MW01125222

MELVILLE HOUSE PUBLISHING
HOBOKEN, NEW JERSEY

©2006 Celia Farber

Book Design: David Konopka

Melville House Publishing
300 Observer Highway
Third Floor
Hoboken, NJ 07030

www.mhpbooks.com

ISBN 10 hc: 1-933633-07-7
ISBN 10 pb: 1-933633-01-8

Library of Congress Cataloging-in-Publication Data

Farber, Celia
Serious adverse events : an uncensored history of AIDS /
Celia Farber.
       p. cm.
   Includes bibliographical references and index.
   ISBN-13: 978-1-993633-07-9 (hc 13 : alk. paper)
   ISBN-10: 1-933633-07-7 (hc 10 : alk. paper)
   ISBN-13: 978-1-933633-01-5 (pb 13 : alk. paper)
   ISBN-10: 1-933633-01-8 (pb 10 : alk. paper)
   1. AIDS (Disease)—History. I. Title.
   RA643.8.F37 2006
   614.5'99392—dc22
                                        2006012086

9   Preface: The Truth Barrier

29   Chapter One: The Passion of Peter Duesberg
65   Chapter Two: "Never Before in the History of Disease"
83   Chapter Three: A Multifactorial Syndrome?
113   Chapter Four: Sins of Omission
143   Chapter Five: The Grey Zone
161   Chapter Six: What About Africa?
183   Chapter Seven: Out of Africa
207   Chapter Eight: The Rebel Genius
221   Chapter Nine: "Only Different in Degree"
229   Chapter Ten: Science Fiction
253   Chapter Eleven: An Era of Openness
275   Chapter Twelve: Out of Control

311   Epilogue

319   Appendix I: World Bank Timeline of Global AIDS Events
331   Appendix II: The Birth of Antibodies Equal Infection

Serious Adverse Events
An Uncensored History of AIDS

"The threat of death hangs over all men and, however disguised it may be, and even if it is sometimes forgotten, it affects them all the time and creates in them a need to deflect death on to others. The formation of baiting crowds answers this need."

Elias Canetti, *Crowds and Power*

Winston Churchill famously said: "The empires of the future are the empires of the mind." This was during his spell of enthusiasm for the implementation of a linga franca used by the Allies called Basic English, a language of only 850 words. George Orwell, during his years at the BBC, was himself interested in Basic, and scholars say it formed the basis of the totalitarian language "Newspeak" in *1984*.

Since April 23, 1984, an empire of the mind has been expanding around our world. It is a simple, terrifying idea, and each mind in which it implants becomes incorporated, as territory, into the empire. It was not really an idea but more of a dictum. Colossally powerful, the dictum was that there was a single sexually transmissible virus that would bring imminent death upon millions of Americans. It was declared during a packed press conference held in Washington, DC—on April 23, 1984—wherein the Secretary of Health and Human Services, Margaret Heckler, declared, "The probable cause of AIDS has been found." She introduced National Cancer Institute virologist Robert Gallo, chief of the Laboratory of Tumor Cell Biology, who explained that he had discovered a collection of retroviral "particles" to be the "probable cause of AIDS." Heckler added that an "AIDS vaccine" could be expected in two years, and that the announcement marked a watershed moment in the "honor roll of American science."

By the next day "probable" had fallen away, and the "novel retrovirus," later named "HIV"—the human immunodeficiency virus—became forever lodged in global consciousness as "the AIDS virus." (The word "probable" was dropped when Lawrence Altman, writing in the *New York Times*, definitively referred to the retrovirus as "the AIDS virus." Altman, the *Times* chief medical reporter, was, at that time, a member of a sub-division of the Centers for Disease Control (CDC) called the Epidemic Intelligence Service (EIS), known as the "medical CIA." He was recruited into the EIS in 1963, six years before he started at the *Times*. Established in 1951, the chief purpose of the EIS was to fan out in various fields, including media, and act as public health activists, promoting the agenda of the CDC, and acting as "its eyes and ears.")

The now famous press conference drop-kicked the world into a new era and marks the beginning of official AIDS history—an event the HHS put on par with NASA's first moon landing.

But others saw it differently. As one AIDS researcher put it to me, "the cause of AIDS was declared by government fiat." Some of the scientists in the audience that day were astonished to the point of speechlessness at Gallo's claims. His viral sample, for a start, was identical to one that had been isolated in Dr. Luc Montagnier's lab at the Pasteur Institute in Paris during the previous year and sent to Gallo for comment. Scientists recognized it— yet nobody said anything. This point has been more rigorously analyzed and proven than any single moment in all of virology, by several investigating committees, journalists—one in particular, John Crewdson, has written hundreds of pages about the sample's appropriation—and, finally, conceded by the U.S. government itself, which, in 1994, quietly settled a long running legal battle with the Pasteur scientists, admitting that they had discovered the virus and that the U.S. therefore owed them millions in HIV test royalties. Montagnier never suggested the virus was the cause of AIDS, but Gallo and the NCI did.

There have been many accounts of the iconic press conference. (I have written the easy, movie version of it myself several times, complete with "flashing bulbs" and "global media" hysteria.) But studying the press conference now through all the threads of history, all the weather systems that led up to this perfect storm, one can see clearly that it was a moment not only of scientific disgrace but a theater of the absurd. If we remove the starchy coverings of the Ambitious Scientist and His Jealous Rivals, the Brave AIDS Activists, The Politicians In Denial, The CDC official twisted into knots of worry because Nobody was Listening, and look at the 1984 press conference starkly, without its casing, we can at last see the strange and disjointed wiring that lay beneath the surface.

Fewer than half (36 percent) of the group of gay male patients on whom Gallo was basing his findings had any sign of the retrovirus at the time. We also know that until that moment in time, retroviruses were considered non-pathogenic, non-cell killing, though of great interest to a generation of "retrovirologists" who had had emerged after the discovery of "reverse transcriptase" in the 1970s.

Gallo claimed "strong evidence of a causative involvement of the virus in AIDS," but it was not a proven scientific fact. Gallo had, at best, identified the retrovirus's presence. He had not shown a causal relationship. Gallo later published four papers in *Science* in the spring of 1984 that form the bedrock of the HIV theory, but looking there, one does not find the fine threads that would explain how he and his colleagues knew HIV "caused" AIDS. This is where the story becomes truly strange. One must wind back to the very first cases of AIDS, in 1981, to understand it.

In 1980, the CDC was trying to recover from the fiasco of what was supposed to have been its shining triumph—the vaccination program against Legionaires Disease, termed the beginning of a "swine flu" epidemic. A few American Legion members had come down with pneumonia at a convention in Philadelphia, and the CDC went into overdrive, insisting that the cause was a microbe found in soil. After mass panic about "swine flu" was spread in the media—reported, as well, by the *Times'* Altman—the CDC developed a research branch devoted to the disease and even a quick vaccine, which was given to fifty million Americans. The vaccine resulted in at least six hundred cases of paralysis and seventy-four deaths. A cascade of lawsuits ensued, and the CDC's chief, who had tried to obscure the vaccine deaths, lost his job. The CDC continued its pursuit of infectious disease causes, because its mission was to stop the *spread* of a disease, ideally through public health measures. Swine flu was, for the CDC, the one that got away. The failure did not cause them to change course, but rather heightened their drive for what they called a "suitable epidemic."

It is assumed that AIDS "broke out," among gay men, but in fact, it was *searched* out. In 1980, Michael Gottlieb, a researcher, at the University of California medical center, "wanted to study the immune system and began scouring the hospital for patients with immune deficiency diseases." He found a case—a man in his early thirties with a yeast infection in his throat and a case of *Pneumocystic cariini* pneumonia. Using a new technology that counted T-cells, a subset of white cells of the immune system, Gottlieb found that his patient had very few. Gottlieb kept searching, and eventually found four more similar cases. Gottlieb excitedly rang up the *New England Journal of Medicine* (*NEJM*) and said: "I've got something that's bigger than Legionaire's. What's the shortest time between submission and publication?" When the *NEJM* refused to rush it into print, Gottlieb turned to the CDC. James Curran, from the agency's Venereal Disease

Division, got the announcement on his desk first, and famously wrote: "Hot stuff. Hot stuff" across it, rushing it into the CDC's weekly newsletter. Soon more cases were reported to the CDC, now with a new symptom: A rare blood vessel tumor called Kaposi's Sarcoma that mostly manifested as purple lesions on the surface of the skin but could also manifest in the internal organs.

The National Institutes of Health (NIH), meanwhile, were burdened by the weight of the utter failure of Nixon's "War on Cancer," which relied on bankrupt theories that included retroviruses as the cause of most cancers. What this meant was that there was a generation of retrovirologists, trained and ready for glory, with no disease to focus on. In the years preceding the first cases of AIDS, federal institutions were filled with frustrated researchers and scientists determined to find viral causes for whatever they could. Chief among them was the National Cancer Institute's Robert Gallo.

Gallo, in an almost comical fashion, spent years trying to find a disease to fit one of his viruses. The model for HIV was established years before it was isolated, as though it had been wished or dreamed into existence. In 1980, Gallo identified his first contender, which he dubbed HTLV, "the first known human retrovirus" (subsequently called HTLV-1). Gallo found his virus concentrated among residents of the Japanese island of Kyushu, as well as in parts of the Caribbean and Africa. Some of them had a type of leukemia called Adult T-cell Leukemia, and that was all Gallo needed to hear. He pushed his theory right into the textbooks, where it remains to this day, despite the total lack of evidence linking HTLV to the illness as a cause.

But here is where the foundations of the new retroviral faith were laid out, preparing the ground for the big one: HTLV was said to cause disease after a several-year-long latency period. The latency period would eventually grow all the way up to an absurd *fifty-five* years, when it was found that the virus is transmitted from mother to child at birth.

In 1982, Gallo added a second virus to his HTLV family, calling it "HTLV-2." Again, he tried to pin it on an obscure form of leukemia, but this time it did not fly. When Gallo, in 1983, "appropriated" Luc Montagnier's LAV virus, later "the AIDS virus," he predictably named it "HTLV-3." Prior to that, he first tried to push HTLV-1 as the cause of AIDS—in other words, the first virus he claimed was connected to AIDS was a leukemia virus. Leukemia is a disease of abundant white cells, while AIDS is a deficiency of white cells.

Decades later, after looking anew at the data, at the reality beneath the roaring fires of the "war on AIDS," serious questions about HIV's ability to cause AIDS have sparked an international science war. It is a war of data, authority, and perception. It is marked by fury, condemnation, and extreme emotion. To this day, the AIDS industry—now a multi-billion dollar operation that has expanded far beyond the CDC and NIH—assails anyone who questions HIV's role in AIDS. This establishment has labeled any critic an "HIV denialist"—a freighted term, of course, meant to slander critics by equating them, in a truly shameless misappropriation, with those who deny the Holocaust. And yet the critics only seem to grow in numbers, cropping up on innumerable websites and in escalating numbers of organizations around the world, from the U.S., to South Africa, to South Korea, Mexico, Brazil, India, Russia, and countless other nations.

This is a book about this larger "AIDS war," what was and is, most simply, an informational war, in the information age, about how and why we think we know what we think we know.

Early on the government's theory about HIV was clearly in crisis: By the late 1980s it was clear that testing positive for HIV was not an immediate death sentence, that living HIV-positive was not only possible but probable. The initial hysteria, however, continued unabated, even after many of the claims of the theory began to give way one after another: that HIV would spread rampantly along lines of "heterosexual sex"; that the drug AZT would "save lives"; that Africa would be "decimated"; that cocktail therapies would eradicate HIV, thus eradicating the problem. And yet all these notions about the epidemic have been largely relegated to obscurity. Or better to say, have been—until now.

The HIV-AIDS hypothesis has entrapped millions of minds since 1984, who were told, in countless languages, the same terrifying message: Those with HIV would, without a doubt, die. They were entrapped by a scientific hypothesis and left no method of escape. HIV-Causes-AIDS-And-Eventual-Death-In-All-Persons-Who-Test-Positive-For-Antibodies was a new type of code unleashed upon the world. It was a code that would fulfill what Canetti calls "the need to deflect death on to others." It did so under the guise of modernity—a new cosmic order brought about by the emerging bio-technologies, chief among which was the "HIV test" itself. Prior to 1984, there were innumerable ways of classifying humans, of drawing lines of race, class, sexuality or whatever else, to ensure that one portion of the world's population could dominate the rest. But none were this sophisticated; none had the appearance of such unquestioned humanity, or, to use a favored term in of the AIDS debate, "compassion."

The HIV-AIDS fear would also blight, in the span of a single day in the spring of 1984, a most fundamental freedom that rarely gets mentioned because it is so self-evident, and that is the *in*ability to see the approaching day of our own death. This was the gift, according to Greek mythology, of Prometheus, who proudly proclaimed of his gift to mortals: "I blinded them to the day of their deaths *so that they would aspire.*"

The ancient Greeks understood this to be a sacred realm, the root of hope itself, of "aspiration," a word which encompasses the very notion of breath.

I have been questioning the surefire death sentence of a positive HIV antibody test since 1987, when as a young reporter I first interviewed a very friendly and affable retroviral scientist named Peter Duesberg for the music magazine *SPIN*. He spelled out, as he has since done with unending patience to countless others, why he had published a scientific paper repudiating the retrovirus HIV as the cause of AIDS or anything else.

Duesberg's story had already been told in the pages of publisher Chuck Ortleb's *New York Native*, a newspaper that doesn't exist anymore—in part because it was boycotted by the AIDS activist organization ACT UP over its "irresponsible" AIDS coverage. I remember being struck by the sight of the *Native*'s cover, in the fall of 1987, when I saw it on a Greenwich Village newsstand. The cover was divided into two images: a photograph of Robert Gallo on one side with the accompanying quote in huge letters, "HIV Kills Like a Truck"; on the other side was his colleague, retroviral titan Peter Duesberg, with his own quote saying, "It's harmless. I wouldn't mind being injected with it." The interview inside was by the *Native*'s star reporter, John Lauritsen. It was intelligent, exhaustive, and very dramatic. I placed a call to Duesberg's office.

Duesberg returned my call at 8 a.m. He was calling from Germany, and he hoped he hadn't woken me. I scrambled to plug in my tape recorder, thanked him for calling back, and started the interview.

To say that I could not have dreamed I would still be writing about him, about this, nearly twenty years later, is an understatement. In 1988, after reporting Duesberg's heresy and other AIDS stories for *SPIN*, I was banished from access to any scientist at the National Institutes of Health. But Duesberg's calm demeanor, and his careful explanation of his thinking about HIV, proved a useful guide to many AIDS stories to come.

Following the publication of that first Duesberg interview, I also received a call from Robert Gallo himself. By contrast, Gallo was intimidating and spoke harshly. "You want to be like Barbara Walters?" he nearly shouted. "How do you think you get there? Not by writing this kind of thing, saying people are wrong. That's not how you make it in this profession." The call lasted well over an hour, and I simply listened. It had no effect on my sense of whether it was right or wrong to pursue the "other side" of this story; it only had an effect on my estimation of these two scientists who had been close friends for years, Gallo and Duesberg. Gallo was passionate, angry, confrontational. Duesberg was calm, gracious, witty. (To represent Gallo's position, *SPIN* published, in the very next issue, an interview with him by science journalist Anthony Liversidge.)

Despite an unrelenting pogrom on his scientific career that sought to blight and silence his unique voice, Duesberg managed, by way of private funders, to secure a good microscope and get back to work studying cells. Over the past ten years has once again rocked a scientific paradigm—this time in cancer genetics, with a theory called the aneuploidy theory of cancer. His success in the field has not, however, made much impact on the public perception of his previous thinking about AIDS, thinking that has been largely discarded and forgotten by mainstream scientists. The two parts of Duesberg's career are still considered separate. This glaring paradox raised an obvious question: What would it mean if the scientist who was "wrong" about AIDS turned out to be "right" about cancer? This book thus begins with the story of Peter Duesberg, the infamous scientist who claims that HIV does not cause AIDS.

The way HIV is assumed to work has been discussed often. It has been claimed that HIV somehow causes cell death—even when it is not present—by remote programmed "suicidal" mechanisms. It is claimed that although HIV does not kill the laboratory T-cells used to manufacture AIDS tests, it does kill T-cells in the human body, even though it infects only a very small proportion of them—Duesberg claims an average of .1 percent. HIV does not sicken or kill chimpanzees, though they do produce antibodies. Unproven hypotheses about the ingenuity of HIV proliferate in the popular and scientific media like the seasonal flu. Seldom do journalists insist on good, hard evidence for these assertions. Those who have received the highest awards in journalism for their AIDS reportage all seem to have made a decision that the only story about AIDS worth reporting was the government's version—the one spinning out from the towers of huge organizations like the National Institutes of Health, the Centers for Disease Control, the World Health Organization, and so forth.

The classical tests of whether or not a microorganism is the cause of infectious disease are known as "Koch's postulates." They state: 1) the microorganism must be found in all cases of the disease; 2) it must be isolated from the host and grown in pure culture; 3) it must reproduce the original disease when introduced into a susceptible host; and 4) it must be found present in the experimental host so infected. Although claims to the contrary have been made, Duesberg maintains that it has never been demonstrated that HIV satisfies all of Koch's postulates. His exhaustive analysis of the peer-reviewed scientific literature has revealed more than 4,000 documented AIDS cases in which there is no trace of HIV or HIV antibodies. This number is significant, because there are strong institutional forces deterring such descriptions and because the vast majority of AIDS cases are never described in formal scientific papers. In fact, most AIDS patients have no active HIV in their systems, because the virus has been neutralized by antibodies. (With most other viral diseases, by the way, the presence of antibodies signals immunity from the disease. Why this is not the case with HIV has never been demonstrated.) Generally speaking, HIV can be isolated only by "reactivating" latent copies of the virus, and then only with extraordinary difficulty. Viral load, one of the clinical markers for HIV, is not a measurement of actual, live virus in the body but the amplified fragments of RNA left over from an infection that has been suppressed by antibodies. Another embarrassment for the HIV hypothesis is the extraordinary latency period between infection and the onset of disease, despite the fact that HIV is biochemically most active within weeks of initial infection. This latency period, which apparently grows with every passing year, enables proponents of the theory to evade Koch's third and fourth postulates.

Prior to the *New York Native*'s first cover story on the Duesberg/Gallo clash, the challenges to the U.S. Government-led theory, though they existed, were obscure and faint. There was, at the time, an underground movement driven by people like the late activist Michael Callen, who emphasized and insisted upon "hope" for what were then called "PWAs"—people living with AIDS. Hope, at that time, was not yet fully demonized, and it resonated with me immediately after meeting Callen in 1987. The "AIDS activist" movement back in those days had dimensionality, and even spirituality, largely thanks to Callen, who resisted what would soon become the harsh, mechanistic, pharma-centric rage of the late '80s ACT UP activism. Callen, who survived with a full-blown AIDS diagnosis for twelve years, always said that *hope* was the single most important element of long-term survival. These were the days when people were deranged with fear and despair, when HIV was said to be transmissible by way of a kiss or a toilet seat.

The HIV-causes-AIDS model was nothing if not mechanistic, and ferociously reductionist. Its net trapped new and emerging technologies. It exploited ancient fears seeded in sex, shame, and death. The net trapped all those who turned up "positive" on an antibody test, a test that has now all but lost all biological meaning and specificity. It was a mark of death, understood at the time as a sure death sentence. In stark terror, millions fled straight into the waiting labyrinth of social stigma, and were willingly treated with a chemotherapy drug that was, then, the most toxic drug ever approved for human use—AZT. Those who could not afford AZT, especially in developing nations, committed suicide, homicide, or tried in innumerable ways to destroy themselves, to live out the terrible prophecy.

This book is about the twenty-year war between those who believed in the death sentence and those who did not. It was, as I say, an informational war—a war of ideas, values, politics, money, power, and the ways that all of those things cast impossible shadows on what was called "irrefutable data," and "overwhelming evidence."

From the ashes of that war, a new narrative is emerging, from the experiences of untold millions who fell into the net, usually by way of a single antibody test, and without any knowledge of the dissent against the official theory. The AIDS war divided those who believed and enacted its every dictum, from those who, very early on, saw a parallel reality, a sister ship loaded with a very different cargo of facts and interpretations. This could only happen at a time when the world was flooded with "information," and yet, mass media gained unsurpassed powers of persuasion. To question the core catechism that HIV was the single and direct cause of AIDS became an act of not only heresy, but grave moral "irresponsibility," finally escalating into open charges of murder. Questioning led to an abatement of fear, and the revolution was *rooted* in fear. HIV-positive women were counseled to abort their fetuses, and even castigated for daring to get pregnant. African men were even circumcised in great numbers, out of the belief that less surface skin meant less territory for HIV to "enter" through.

I have taken the phrase "The Truth Barrier" from the title of a 1978 collection by the Swedish poet Tomas Transtromer to invoke the membrane where "truth" struggles to reconcile itself with a disturbed world. Transtromer's frequent use of the word "truth" is the equivalent of nature itself. In many poems Transtromer describes how easily "truth" breaks when we try too hard to catch it, possess it, personify it. A "scientific truth" is after all a secret of nature, not of man. It always rises to the surface and confronts the world. In the poem "Preludes," he writes: "Two truths draw nearer each other. One comes from inside, one comes from outside, and where they meet we have a chance to see ourselves. He who notices what is happening cries despairingly: 'Stop! Whatever you like, if only I can avoid knowing myself.'"

Beneath the industrial, social roar of all we mean when we say "AIDS" is yet another of nature's secrets that man presumes to have unlocked. My one certainty is that something very critical is working itself out here, through this epic scientific clash. Does HIV cause AIDS? I don't know if it does or it does not—I'm not really equipped to know. The story I have tried to tell, and which this book explores, is the story not of my own beliefs about science (I am not a scientist) but of the epic *human* drama between those who say yes and those who say no to this question. It's part of "what happened." But it's not only news—it's Shakespearian. And I for one really want to know how it's going to end.

Scientific curiosity, which Einstein called "holy," is alive and well. That is the good news. It survives in the circuitry of minds not driven by fear, and despite the systemic and near maniacal persecution of those who think differently from prevailing dogma. Whatever the truth may turn out to be, it is something that involves us all, moves through us, from inside and from outside, drawing nearer and slipping away.

On any given story, a dominant narrative takes shape, and journalists form a herd around it. Stories that pertain to government, as AIDS does, are strictly controlled and censored. That's a given. Journalists who don't follow the herd are swiftly cut off from access to what they call "sources." This book is thus subtitled "an uncensored history," because it depends almost entirely on sources that have been censored—most especially by their own fear to speak out—and almost none on sources in government.

Much of what appears in this volume was first published elsewhere, and it retains its contemporaneous tone here. Where possible, material has been updated to reflect new information, but many of the stories included here are reprinted as they were originally published.

For facts that fall outside the scope of this book, a rough guide to the accepted history of global AIDS events, including epidemiological estimates of the AIDS epidemic, is provided in Appendix I; the timeline was composed for the World Bank report "Committing to Results: Improving the Effectiveness of HIV/AIDS Assistance." A more controversial history of the way in which antibodies to HIV began signaling HIV infection is reprinted as Appendix II; this timeline was composed by Rodney Richards, a former employee of Amgen, now the world's largest biotech company, who worked with Abbott Laboratories on the development of the ELISA HIV test.

Chapter Two, "Never Before in the History of Disease," was originally published in *SPIN* (August 1988).

The research and quotations that comprise Chapter Three, "A Multifactorial Syndrome?," was also first published in *SPIN*. I first explored the topic of co-factors in the April 1988 issue; I wrote about and interviewed Michael Callen for the June 1988, April 1991, and April 1994 issues. I reported about the question of mycoplasma in the September 1990 issue.

Much of Chapter Four, "Sins of Omission," was researched, written, and published in *SPIN* in 1989 at the very peak of pro-AZT hysteria, during a time in which the drug was credited with being "the only drug" that could "save people's lives." At the time of its publication, *SPIN* took out a full-page ad in the *New York Times* noting: "Before you take AZT again, read the November issue of *SPIN*." My coverage of the ACTG 076 trial was originally published in *Mothering* (September/October 1998).

Chapter Five, "The Grey Zone," is drawn from a number of pieces I wrote about HIV-negative AIDS, including features first published in *SPIN* in October 1992 and April 1996.

My reporting on the AIDS epidemic in Africa, which is considerably updated here, is accompanied by the long piece, "Out of Africa," which was first published in *SPIN* in March and April of 1993. Chapter Six draws on much of the research I did about the predicted heterosexual AIDS epidemic in the U.S. and first published as "Fatal Distractions" in the June 1992 issue of *SPIN*.

My profile of Kary Mullis, "The Rebel Genius," is drawn from conversations that were first published in the June 1992 and July 1994 issues of *SPIN*.

My writing about protease inhibitors was first seen in *SPIN* as a short feature, "The End of The End?," in April 1997. In March 2000, I published "Science Fiction" in *Gear*; it has been significantly updated here.

I first reported on the scandal at ICC in New York City for the online magazine *Red Flags*. Chapter Eleven also includes the research and writing I did about AIDS activist organizations in "Money Changes Everything," which was published in *SPIN*, September 1992.

"Out of Control" was first published, in a slightly different form, in *Harper's Magazine* (March 2006).

"Peter Duesberg is a man of extraordinary energy, unusual honesty, enormous sense of humor, and a rare critical sense. This critical sense often makes us look twice, then a third time, at a conclusion many of us believed to be foregone. . . . an extraordinary scientist. . . . "

—Robert Gallo at the National Cancer Institute, 1984

The sun is hot on my head as I cross the campus of the University of California at Berkeley, looking for Donner Lab, the university's oldest science building, where virologist Peter Duesberg has recently been relocated. It's early spring, 2004, and it's been a few years since I last visited the campus.

I stop two students and ask for directions. They pull out a campus map; they've never heard of it. Finally they just give me their map and wish me luck. Eventually I find it. To say that it is on the periphery of the campus is an understatement: It is practically in the woods.

The Berkeley campus is looking very grand these days, its important halls adorned with oblong hedges clipped to perfection. It's very quiet. Hard to imagine this having once been a bastion of radical protest. Thanks to large donations from two pharmaceutical companies, Berkeley's biology facilities are undergoing extensive renovation. There are bulldozers here and there, and near Donner Lab is a huge gaping hole where a building has just been demolished. In the distance, I spot Peter Duesberg weaving on his bicycle past the bulldozers on his way into the lab. In the heat of the sun, it seems to me that their jaws might just reach down and snap him up, putting a quick, merciful end to the nearly twenty-year battle between the Establishment and the troublesome scientist.

In the years since Duesberg, by invitation, wrote a paper in a prominent journal detailing his critique of the then half-formed theory that retroviruses caused human cancers, and adding almost as an afterthought that the garden-variety retrovirus HIV could by no means cause a "disease" such as AIDS, he's been facing bulldozers almost wherever he goes. Reviled by the AIDS establishment, de-funded by the NIH, ostracized and all but exiled within the university where he is a tenured professor, Duesberg was invited back to his native Germany in 1996 to resume his work on cancer. During this time, commuting bi-annually between Mannheim and Berkeley, he formulated and tested a theory that has brought a new glitter to his complicated name. Some cancer-theorists say it's nothing short of the genetic answer to cancer. Others say it is at least part of the answer. It's lucky for Peter Duesberg that AIDS and cancer are distinct fields; his detractors in the AIDS field have made clear that they want him sunk to the bottom of the deepest sea, even if the answer to cancer goes with him.

In what is shaping up to be a denouement of Shakespearean proportions, it looks as though America's most controversial biologist may be poised for resurrection. When *Scientific American* recently published a lengthy article on our current understanding of cancer genetics, Duesberg's picture was on the timeline for 1999, the year he formalized and published his new theory. At Berkeley, he recently broke—by nearly twofold—the record for undergrad students applying for research assistantships with him. Breaking a seventeen-year embargo against inviting Duesberg anywhere, to address anyone, the National Cancer Institute (NCI) has invited him to their headquarters to speak on cancer. And a first biography, *Oncogenes, Aneuploidy, and AIDS: A Scientific Life and Times of Peter Duesberg,* by Harvey Bialy, has been published. Still, at Berkeley, where his department remains overtly, almost flamboyantly hostile, Duesberg had to appeal to the chancellor for a so-called merit pay increase, which usually comes automatically to professors of his stature. After the dean of the Division of

Biological Sciences had denied him a merit increase for three years based on the department's recommendation that his work was "not of high significance," the merit pay increase was finally granted in 2004, by a dean from the Physical Sciences Division.

If Duesberg's name sounds familiar, it's because he has been branded in mainstream media as the virologist who is wrong about HIV. His name entered the popular culture in the late 1980s pre-stamped with wrongness. You knew he was wrong before you knew what he had said in the first place. It wasn't just that he was wrong, he was wrong to have even posed the question about which he was declared spectacularly wrong. He was wrong to have created an air-pocket for the public in which to even *think* about whether the HIV-AIDS hypothesis was right or wrong, because prior to him no such space exsisted, certainly no language. And this was his real crime. At a time of unprecedented social and sexual terror, Duesberg was said to be killing people with his very ideas—in this case a dissenting argument that HIV was not, in fact, the cause of AIDS.

When Peter Duesberg first questioned the HIV hypothesis, authorities were claiming HIV would wipe out one quarter of the U.S. population in three years. Duesberg had, in effect, created a template for a question that was supposed to be unthinkable, and which, to the AIDS industry, was not only preposterous, it was virtually obscene: Does HIV really *cause* AIDS?

He did so in the form of a lengthy, highly technical paper. It was a paper that, in the words of his biographer Harvey Bialy, had "disastrous professional consequences" for Duesberg and "sealed his scientific fate for almost two decades."

At the age of fifty Duesberg became one of the youngest inductees of the U.S. National Academy of Sciences for his pioneering work in the 1970s that defined the first cancer genes and mapped the genetic structure of retroviruses. He has argued since 1987 that HIV is not pathogenic, i.e., not capable of killing cells, i.e., not the cause of AIDS. His case is amply documented, but not surprisingly, still unfamiliar to most people. This is not a "debate," it is a huge chasm between two sets of conclusions reached by looking at the same data. Each side thinks the other side is dead-wrong, and there has been little or no synthesis or compromise reached in the years since Duesberg's paper.

The cadre of scientists who signed a petition in 1991 stating they agreed with Duesberg and wanted the case re-opened included three Nobel Laureates and 600 PhDs. Still, the standard paragraph in any article you'll ever read about Duesberg will say that no "respectable scientist" agrees with him and that he as been "refuted."

Duesberg had been at the very top of his field when the trouble began. Suddenly a furious cyclone moved in, and he was openly and unceremoniously stripped of everything: Government funding, grad students, a proper lab, invitations to conferences. But for all the recent signs of rehabilitation, Duesberg remains 100 percent cut off from NIH funding, despite continuing to submit grant proposals regularly, now exclusively on cancer. Prior to 1987, he was one of the most generously funded scientists in the nation and never had a grant turned down. Since 1987, he has submitted a total of twenty-three grant proposals to non-private agencies, and every single one has been rejected. In orthodox AIDS circles, his name still triggers a symphony of emotions from distain to fury.

In a recent documentary, *The Other Side of AIDS,* there is a remarkable scene in which Canadian MD Mark Wainberg, president of the International AIDS Society, the world's largest organization of AIDS researchers and clinicians, angrily calls for Duesberg and others who "attempt to dispel the notion that HIV is the cause of AIDS," to be "brought up on trial," calling such people "perpetrators of death." He goes on to say that he would hope the U.S. Constitution could be re-written to accommodate such arrests.

In the film, Wainberg's large face grows pale with fury as he realizes that the interviewer himself is sympathetic towards Duesberg's ideas and is thus one of the so-called AIDS "dissidents." Wainberg unleashes a lengthy tirade, accusing all HIV skeptics of wanting "millions of people in Africa and elsewhere" to get HIV and die, and finally, he shouts: "*I suggest to you that Peter Duesberg is the closest thing we have on this planet to a scientific psychopath.*"

"Are we clear that what you are going to do is present things as they are?" said Harvey Bialy, Duesberg's scientific biographer, in a deep, stern voice over the phone from his office in Cuernavaca, Mexico. "I'm not going to answer questions about *why* these things are, only *how* they came to be. Speculations about motives don't interest me. You can't document motives. You *think* you know who this man is and what he said, but you don't. That's the starting point for your reader."

Bialy, a Berkeley-educated molecular biologist and friend of Duesberg since 1966 is a longstanding HIV-AIDS critic in his own right and was the founding scientific editor of *Nature BioTechnology*, a sister journal to *Nature*. His book, *Oncogenes, Aneuploidy, and AIDS: A Scientific Life and Times of Peter Duesberg,* is an extremely detailed history of the papers, review articles, and letters that Duesberg published between 1983 and 2003 and the responses they generated. Baily writes in airless, acute prose untouched by any of the usual attitudes, convictions, and emotions that have colored virtually ever word written or uttered about Duesberg since the fateful year of 1987.

Perhaps the most striking quality of the book is that he writes of Duesberg as simply a scientist. Not as a disgraced, fallen scientist, but a scientist—period. The book does not disparage him, nor does it elevate him; it simply records Duesberg's scientific arc through the three fields of study on which he has had an almost immeasurable impact: Oncogenes, Aneuploidy, and AIDS. Let's shorten that to: Cancer and AIDS.

In sharp contrast to his controlled prose, Bialy's temperament is volatile and acerbic. He doesn't particularly wish to be interviewed and is indignant about all the non-science that has clouded Duesberg's biological oeuvre since the mid-1980s, a time he refers to as "celebrity-culture" science.

I asked him why he wrote this book—a project that took four years.

"It was when I read Peter's third aneuploidy paper in 1999 that I was persuaded he had nailed the initiating event in carcinogenesis. Peter has found the genetic basis for cancer. The most immediate application of it will be early diagnosis. So when aneuploidy, or genetic instability as it is sometimes called, gets reincarnated as the dominant theoretical explanation for the genesis of cancer, Peter Duesberg will be recognized as a major contributor. I wanted to make sure that his contributions were not swept aside or ignored."

"Scientifically," he adds almost as an afterthought, "cancer is still an interesting question. AIDS has not been an interesting question for ten years."

"Why do you say that?"

His voice rises. "Doesn't the book demonstrate very clearly that scientifically, nothing happened between 1994 and 2003? Zero. Absolutely nothing except one wrong epidemiological prediction after another, one failed poisonous drug after another. 0.000.000 cured, as AmFAR [The American Foundation for AIDS Research] likes to remind us in their never-ending fundraising. There is still no vaccine. They've got nothing to show for twenty years and 50+ billion U.S. taxpayer dollars. Nada, nothing. HIV/AIDS has been a total scientific and medical failure. We've turned virology inside out and upside down to accommodate this bullshit hypothesis. It's enough to make me use indecorous language."

I imagine Mark Wainberg's livid face, and imagine how it would look if he heard *this* conversation.

"Look, AIDS is a political thing, and Peter's stuck in it. I show in the book how he came to get stuck, but other than that there's nothing to discuss anymore."

To Bialy, in the end, the critical point was that science is amoral and should be.

"Peter is not a *good* scientist, a *bad* scientist, a *mediocre* scientist, a *great* scientist, a *brilliant* scientist, or an unstable one for that matter. If you must use an adjective to characterize him, use classical. Peter is a *classical* molecular biologist. He is only interested in rigorously testing dueling hypotheses. The twin pillars, AIDS and Oncogenes, both are crumbling because of the questions he put into motion."

Peter Duesberg is bent over a metal tray with twelve Petri dishes filled with pink gel, squirting each carefully with the tip of a long thin nozzle. He hears me come in and without looking up he starts to talk. "These are breast cancer cells that have been treated with chemotherapy." He leans in closer and his cadence slows. "Fortunately... this time, it is in the Petri dish and not... in somebody's... body."

He finishes, pushes his goggles up on his forehead, and darts over to the microwave at the other side of the lab where he is heating two cups of green tea. "You want some?" he says. "It's good stuff." He moves very fast and he talks almost constantly, punctuating serious scientific arguments with a kind of absurdist black humor, all in a fairly pronounced German accent. Many people may be anguishing about what was done to him, but he himself doesn't seem too upset. He jokes about it. Remarking on his current position, in what he calls "the semi-outhouse" of Donner Lab, he tells me about his private funders, who keep him in business. "It's small compared to NIH grants but not bad for what I'm doing; it's perfect terrorist science. You can do it almost undercover. All you need is a belt and a little dynamite and a microscope." He laughs and hands me a mug swirling with tea leaves and puts a long, thin glass "Pasteur Pipette" in it for me to stir with. "Those are disposable," he says. "Don't worry, there's no radioactivity on them."

He sits on a stool, stirs his tea and says, distractedly, "I really think we may have found it."

His lab assistant, Ruhong Li, who's been quietly peering into a microscope looks up for a moment. Li has been working closely with Duesberg since 1990; the silent, sober, fastidious counter-part to Duesberg's prankster persona.

What he means by "it" is the one thing all cancer cells he has ever studied have in common. For the past three decades, genetic cancer theory has assumed that cancer results from one or several gene mutations, in so-called oncogenes. Every human being has about 25,000 genes strung like beads along the strings of forty-six chromosomes. For most of the last century, cancer researchers have been focusing on the beads. Now the focus is shifting to the strings.

Duesberg has revived, honed, and mathematically formalized a view of cancer causation that was first articulated in 1914 by another German geneticist; it's called the aneuploidy theory of cancer. It posits that cancer is caused not by a series of genetic mutations, as current dogma holds, but by a misfiring in the critical moment that chromosomes divide.

Duesberg has reinvigorated the discovery first made by Theodor Boveri in 1914—that all cancers have chromosomal abnormalities: The numbers of chromosomes in the cell are incorrect, and there are broken, enlarged, and fused chromosomes, as though mashed by faulty machinery. Boveri used doubly fertilized sea urchin eggs to make cells with one and half the normal number of chromosomes—they were tumors. He concluded that cancer was a result of excess or disturbed chromosomes.

Duesberg has further provided, in a series of experiments, functional evidence for his hypothesis that places aneuploidy at the center of the genetic tragedy that is cancer, while relegating gene mutation to the deepest wings. Many cancer researchers are willing to follow him up to the point where he discards mutant gene theory, arguing that both are an important part of the picture. But Duesberg, despite isolating the first oncogene (cancer gene) in the early 1970s, has been arguing since the early 1980s that, in general, mutant genes don't cause cancer, and as he added almost incidentally, neither do retroviruses.

"The basis of speciation is changing the content and the number of chromosomes," says Duesberg. "Cancer is essentially a failed speciation. It's not mutation. Cancer is a *species*. A really bad breast, lung, or prostate cancer has seventy, eighty, or more chromosomes. Those are the real bad guys—they're way outside our species. But it's a rare kind of species that as a parasite is more successful in its host than the normal host cell is."

"All mammals," he continues, "have the same kit of genes. So how do you go from a bat in the air to a whale cruising underwater for days at a time? Well, by regrouping the same old genes in different sets of chromosomes."

Duesberg maintains that 100 percent of solid tumors are aneuploid. "We're not the first to see this. Boveri was. But we're a close second, with a hiatus of eighty years," he says. "Boveri had a great theory, but even then they started attacking him because they were all for mutation. Genes were the sexy thing. That's the smallest unit in biology, the atom of biology. So they wanted it to be genes and they still do. Chromosomes, as [Nobel laureate Michael] Bishop once said in a speech, was 'something little old ladies could see peering through a microscope.' They're so obvious."

In January of 2004, Duesberg hosted a conference on the role of aneuploidy in cancer, inviting fifty cancer researchers from all corners of the world. Seventy showed up. They included such luminaries as NCI's head of Cancer Genomics, Thomas Ried, Gert Auer from the Karolinska Institute in Stockholm, and Walter Giaretti, who heads Italy's equivalent of the NCI.

The conference was, by all accounts, a great success. Perhaps partly because the cancer establishment is much older than the AIDS establishment, an open discussion about the problems of mutant gene theory was possible. The discussion, according to one of the organizers, Dr. David Rasnick, one of Duesberg's closest collaborators, centered on the fact that, mathematically and logically, a few mutant genes can't cause cancer. Rasnick likened the problem of mutant gene theory to literature: Let's say the whole genome is a biological dictionary, divided into volumes called chromosomes, then the life of a cell is a Shakespearean drama. "If one were to misspell a word here and there, in Hamlet for example, it wouldn't affect it much. But you could reduce it to gibberish if you deleted entire portions of text, copied others and shuffled them around at random. That's what aneuploidy does to the cell."

As Duesberg explains it, when a cell divides, it doubles its chromosome number, briefly, and all the chromosomes line up in the middle of the two future cells. "The pairs of chromosomes are lined up in the middle," Duesberg explains, "like soccer teams before they blow the whistle and start the game." At either end are two tiny cables, one attached to each pair of chromosomes. When life begins, each one pulls from its side and the chromosome are forever parted. "Mechanically, it's an unbelievable achievement," says Duesberg. "It almost always happens perfectly, and everybody gets one half."

But sometimes it fails. The only chromosomal failure nature lets slip in humans is one extra chromosome, number 21, which produces Down's Syndrome. People with Down's Syndrome are mildly aneuploid in their whole cellular system, and they are thirty times more likely to develop cancer during their lifetime than other people. Every carcinogen Duesberg's lab has tested (asbestos, hormones, hydrocarbons, etc.) also causes aneuploidy.

Many cancer researchers agree that aneuploidy is "important." What they differ on is how important: Is it sufficient by itself to explain cancer, and do you find it in all cancers? Duesberg and Li are insistent that to date, nobody has produced a diploid (chromosomally normal) cancer cell.

MIT cancer researcher Robert Weinberg published a paper in *Nature* in 1999 claiming to show that three so-called cancer genes were sufficient to convert a normal diploid human cell into a cancer cell. Were it true, it would have been functional proof at last for the long prevailing theory that gene mutations cause cancer. Suspecting that the cells were aneuploid, Duesberg asked Weinberg to send the cell lines so he could study them. "To his credit, he sent them," Duesberg says. But when Duesberg and Li analyzed the cells using their state of the art technology, they found that every single one was aneuploid. They published their findings in *Cancer Research*. Weinberg's team replied in a letter to the journal, saying that Duesberg's lab must have somehow contaminated the cells after receiving them. Subsequently, renowned tumor virologist Hidesaburo Hanafusa tried to repeat Weinberg's findings as well, but all the cancer cells he generated turned out to be aneuploid, too.

The *Scientific American* article broke the current state of cancer-think into four essential camps: Standard dogma, Modified Dogma, Early Instability, and All-aneuploidy. Those who have followed Duesberg's scientific arc were not at all surprised to see Duesberg take the most uncompromising position—all aneuploidy.

Many experts in the field disagree with him, of course, but they all disagree from some place on the aneuploidy *spectrum,* which ranges from: it's important but not causative; to it's very important but not causative; to the Duesberg position, which is that it is the very engine of cancer.

Thomas Ried, chief of the Section of Cancer Genomics at the NCI, attended Duesberg's conference, and has been focusing on aneuploidy himself for most of his career. I visited him in his lab at the NCI in the spring of 2004. He made the case that far from being controversial, aneuploidy theory has been well known and incorporated into American cancer research for many years. He shrugged. "Duesberg is right. But it's not like a big paradigm shift. If anyone had looked at chromosome aberrations in cancer and not realized that it's important, he or she would have been stupid. The director of the NCI called me up not long ago and said, 'I would like to discuss aneuploidy.' We've invited Duesberg here to give a talk on it."

That's odd, considering that the NCI still refuses to fund Duesberg. He has submitted dozens of grant proposals to study aneuploidy, and one of the most influential cancer researchers in the country, Bert Vogelstein, Clayton Professor of Oncology at Johns Hopkins Medical School, even wrote a letter urging them to reconsider, which was reprinted in Bialy's book. "I agree with him that aneuploidy is an essential part of cancer," he wrote. "Duesberg continues to have a major impact on this burgeoning area of research, through his careful experimental observations as well as through his thoughtful reviews and critiques of the subject. There is no question that he is a world leader in this field of investigation."

Ried deflected the question of why or whether NCI might fund Duesberg, saying only that he hadn't personally reviewed any of his grant proposals, assuring me that if he wrote a good one he would be considered for funding in the future.

I asked Ried if he had hesitated before accepting Duesberg's invitation to speak at his conference. "No," he said simply. Then he got up and pulled a copy of a book by Theodor Boveri from a shelf. He tossed it on the table. He smiled. "Duesberg won't get jailed for talking about aneuploidy. Actually I was curious to meet with him and discuss this with him. I don't understand why he has to polarize the issue so much though. He says gene mutations don't play a role. I disagree with that. It doesn't serve a scientific purpose to say that."

"Peter Duesberg is one of the top aneuploidy researchers in the country," said William Brinkley, vice president and dean, Graduate School of BioMedical Sciences, Baylor College of Medicine. "I don't agree with him that gene mutations don't play any role, but he's a stellar scientist. I cite him all the time, and I was pleased to attend his conference on aneuploidy." Although Brinkly did add, "A lot of people have said to me, 'Don't cite that guy. Don't go there.' Because of the associations with his name."

"I think he's a very creative scientist, but he has blinders on," says Dr. John Murnane, a cancer researcher at UCSF, who also attended Duesberg's conference. "I don't have anything against Peter, but I do think he made a mistake in not being more careful about the HIV issue. It had so many social implications and I think it would have been more responsible if he said he thinks people should avoid HIV."

I asked him if he considered not attending the conference because of Duesberg's name. "Honestly? Yes. I thought about, what if somebody sees my name on this list. But then I decided to go anyway."

"His ideas are very brilliant," says Walter Giaretti, director of Italy's National Cancer Institute, who also came to the conference. "I still think gene mutations are important. I'm a partisan of both theories together, but we confronted each other in a passionate, beautiful way. This is the most important question in oncology. It's difficult. 99.99 percent of the research is on gene mutations and so we have to cope with this. Not just give up. Anyway, it was a very stimulating conference."

George Miklos, director of Secure Genetics in Sydney, Australia, departs strongly from the compromise position that keeps a role for mutant genes. "I read Duesberg's 1997 *PNAS* [*Proceedings of the National Academy of Sciences*] paper on aneuploidy. I read it, I put it down, and I said 'This guy has got it right.' It was a revelation and it was instantaneous."

Miklos reviewed Bialy's book in *Nature BioTechnology* and gave it extremely high praise. "I actually saw Bialy's book on Duesberg as not really being about cancer or AIDS at all. I saw it as being a book about maintaining standards. It's following in the tradition, the German tradition actually, of people like Gunther

Stent and Max Delbruck. Duesberg comes from that tradition, and that's why I get so passionate about him. He's put a stake in the sand and said, 'Look, you cross that line and you're lost. You've lost everything. Not just how you do your science but how you maintain your standards everywhere.' That's why it's so important. Once you make that first little step on your downward slope there is no way you can come back."

Miklos, who comes from an aristocratic Hungarian background, views the Duesberg story as an inevitable result of the decline in rules of scientific code and conduct, beginning in the "modern" era of the late 1960s. "Science used to be a gentlemanly pursuit, and the values of the old aristocracy were all about *form*. It's not who wins or loses, it's how you play the game. That's all gone now, and America is of course a brutally competitive society, and the only value is winning, no matter how you go about it."

"Among the values we were inculcated with was the value of looking at the data without looking at the person. We were taught not to think ad hominem, because that was a real threat to science. Duesberg's name didn't ring any bells when I read that first paper. His name of course had been highlighted because of AIDS, but that was always a mess, and this was a totally different field. It was the data itself that came crashing down on me when I read it.

"What must be conceded, no matter how you feel about Duesberg, is that he is the father of modern *experimental* aneuploidy theory. Instead of just saying I see a cancer cell and I find mutations in it or aneuploidy or some other bloody thing and I conclude therefore that they are the cause, Duesberg got down and dirty and provided the experimental proof. He physically took cells and applied the perturbations to them. He physically made the cells aneuploid, 100 percent of the time, by adding carcinogens.

That was the 1997 paper. Then the other killer experiment was in 2001, when you take the pressure of the drugs off them, those cells revert to being non-resistant. This can't be explained by gene mutations. It's impossible."

Duesberg and I walk around the corner to his office, where he kneels down and pulls out the 1987 *Cancer Research* paper, the one that started it all. It turns out the very first reference cited is Theodor Boveri. "I was really a free thinker at that time more than I knew," he says, and shows me that the paper contains early contours of the aneuploidy theory.

Together with virologist Peter Vogt, Duesberg isolated the first supposed cancer gene (oncogene) from a very rare kind of retrovirus. But Duesberg himself had doubts about the relevance of these rare viral oncogenes to cause human cancers. These doubts would grow, as doubts tend to grow in Duesberg's mind, to the point of critical urgency. Peter Vogt hasn't spoken to him in twenty years.

"I was a hero. They loved it. Great idea! Every MD around the globe took his favorite cancer and looked for oncogenes. They awarded several Nobel prizes for this stuff, without ever proving it really happened, that genes caused cancer. [Michael] Bishop and [Harold] Varmus became the kings of cancer and all the rest of it. The trouble was none of these guys bothered to clone them and put them in normal (diploid) cells and see if they're transforming, which was what I was trained to do with viruses."

Before the bio-tech boom of the mid-1980s, Duesberg's fastidiousness and insistence on functional evidence were not only tolerated, they earned him a reputation as a fierce scientific debater with whom one did not want to tangle. But by the time AIDS appeared, these qualities would be recast as "obsessive to the point of pathological" by some of his former friends.

The retroviral-cancer field and the retrovirus-AIDS field, both powered by the emerging biotech industries, were no places for doubts, but Duesberg was all about doubts. More accurately: He was all about transparent data, at a time when biology was becoming increasingly opaque. "If the gene would do what it is said to do it would be very simple," he says. "You would take the gene out of the cancer cell, put it in a normal cell, and get a cancer cell. But that has never worked, despite Nobel prizes and twenty years of mutation-cancer. There is no functional proof for a cancer gene."

By the late 1980s, Duesberg concluded that he and his colleagues had gotten tangled up in a whole lot of complex ideas about retroviruses and oncogenes that were leading nowhere. "So I hit the library," he said, "and aneuploidy was everywhere. In my mind I was already conditioned to think about aneuploidy because there you have thousands of genes changing species. I was thinking, as soon as I finish this AIDS thing I have to go look at that."

But the "AIDS thing" instead crashed in on him and shattered his scientific career.

When, in 1987, he wrote the paper in *Cancer Research*, he unleashed the fury of the NIH that had already been brewing for some time. It became one of the most sensational, vicious, and personal battles in the history of modern science.

Back in 1986, the waters were still calm. Duesberg received a special NIH cancer fellowship, as well as the highly coveted Outstanding Investigator Grant, which is reserved for the top scientists in the country and designed to let them push the boundaries of scientific thought. He was also inducted into the elite National Academy of Sciences, the Hall of Fame for scientists.

Then came the 1987 paper, and all hell broke loose. Its title was hardly incendiary: "Retroviruses as Carcinogens and Pathogens: Expectations and Reality." In it, Duesberg argues against the ideas that retrovirus cause leukemia, other cancers, and finally AIDS. Retroviruses, Duesberg reminded his colleagues in this paper, are not "cytocidal," meaning not cell-killers. However you may feel about the veracity of the HIV hypothesis, it is certainly true to say that to accept it, one has to accept a sudden and total reversal of what was held to be true about retroviruses until April of 1984.

The *Cancer Research* paper is, for the purposes of the layperson, essentially a sweeping reality check against overblown claims for retroviruses, written by the man who at that point in time was said to know them better than anybody. (Robert Gallo once noted that "Peter Duesberg knows more about retroviruses than any man alive.")

But shortly after the *Cancer Research* paper appeared, a memo was sent out from the office of the secretary of Health and Human Services with the words "MEDIA ALERT" that castigated the NIH for allowing the paper to have been published in the first place. "The article apparently went through the normal pre-publication process and should have been flagged at NIH," it read. "This obviously has the potential to raise a lot of controversy. . . . I have already asked NIH public affairs to start digging into this." The memo listed the few media outlets that had covered Duesberg's review and cited a few journalists by name that it promised to check up on.

The notion that the NIH expects to vet every scientific paper in every cancer journal is surprising to people who think of science in the old fashioned, romantic way. But to anybody who knows the system it is no surprise at all. The NIH maintains tight control over the ideas that emanate from U.S. government science, and that control extends to the media, who are rewarded and punished in accordance with their suspension of curiosity.

The NIH and all its branches are not only part of the "government," they are part of the U.S. military. Public Health has its roots in the military; the NIH began during World War I as an organization that focused solely on the health of soldiers. This remained its core mandate through World War II, after which it expanded to become a more sweeping public health institution. Still, top NIH scientists hold military rank—the only openly stated one being the Surgeon General.

The NIH, UC Berkeley, the respectable science press, and, needless to say, the world's many thousands of AIDS organizations, choked on Duesberg as if a bone had lodged in its throat. Ironically, though, his achievements and reputation had lodged him deep in the system; it would take a while for them to spit him out.

The Outstanding Investigator Grant Duesberg had received was designed to allow elite scientists to focus on their work with the cushion of a seven year grant, the idea being that they shouldn't spend precious time on grant-seeking. So the NIH was unable, legally, to close the spigot of funds to Duesberg until 1993. But when Duesberg's grant came up for renewal, he had the proverbial "snowball's chance in summer," as Bialy put it. The review committee included one AIDS researcher who had financial ties to the company that made AZT, a drug Duesberg continually criticized for its extreme toxicity, and one who had mothered a child by the scientist who spawned the HIV-AIDS hypothesis, Robert Gallo. Three reviewers never even read the proposal. Duesberg was doomed. The U.S. government unceremoniously pulled the plug and would never again give him a single research dollar. He went from being among the government's most highly funded scientists to being completely cut off. A kind of anti-Duesbergism swept the field and grew to a near-frenzy. A 1988 interview with Robert

Gallo about Duesberg was laced with furious and even profane cursing. "Cock and horseshit, baloney! HIV kills like a truck!" he hollered. "HIV would kill Clark Kent!" This was in the earliest days of HIV fear, when it was said to be not so much a mysterious virus as a potent, muscular cell-killer that ate T-cells like Pac Man. It is impossible to trace where this belief came from. Retroviruses are mass-produced in cell lines, often in the very T-cells HIV was said to be destroying

In other fields, such as gene therapy, it is axiomatic that retroviruses are the ideal carriers for genetic materials, because they "don't kill cells." Incredibly, this is where the so-called HIV debate first forked in 1987, and where the camps remain bitterly divided to this day. Do retrovirus kill cells or don't they? Duesberg's quip, at the time, was that he wouldn't mind being injected with HIV—so long as the sample didn't come from Gallo's lab.

The shock was palpable, and the first reaction was a kind of queasy silence. The official position became that to address Duesberg's arguments was itself wrong, because it deflected valuable time away from the business of "saving lives," as well as lent credence to dangerous nonsense. AIDS organizations posted warnings about Duesberg and the "denialists" on their websites. Project Inform's Martin Delaney campaigned to get journalists who interviewed Duesberg fired. He didn't have to write many letters, because very few wanted to write about Duesberg. Those who did were quickly set straight. The director of the National Institute of Allergy and Infectious Diseases, Anthony Fauci, tried to make sure Duesberg never appeared on national television by intimidating producers who in some cases had already booked Duesberg and flown him to New York.

A few times he was cancelled within an hour of air-time, only to turn on the TV and see Anthony Fauci himself on the show. Hostility against Duesberg enveloped the administration at Berkeley where his colleagues found themselves unable to expel him, because he had tenure.

He was in short order "dis-invited" from all scientific conferences, and colleagues even declared that they would refuse to attend any conference that included Duesberg. His university dissuaded all grad students from working with him, telling them that it would destroy their careers—so he lost his grad students. He was banished also from publishing in the scientific press, most theatrically by *Nature*'s editor John Maddox. Maddox even wrote a bizarre editorial stating that Duesberg should not be entitled to the standard scientific publishing practice of "Right of Reply" in the wake of frequent attacks on Duesberg being published in *Nature*. This written record is rendered in vivid in Bialy's book. Even the National Academy's journal, *Proceedings of the National Academy of Sciences,* where members are entitled to unfettered access, canceled a Duesberg paper on HIV after he spent over a year revising and re-submitting it to meet their various editing requests.

Those who tried to help Duesberg were themselves attacked, and, in any case, it did no good. The virologist Harry Rubin (himself a member of the Academy) intervened on Duesberg's behalf to try to get the *Proceedings* article published, but it was to no avail. Duesberg's paper in 1992 became the second one in *Proceedings'* 128-year history to be blocked from publication. (The other was written by Linus Pauling.)

Duesberg's name became degraded to the point where it became a means of career advancement to debase him.

Elias Canetti, in *Crowds and Power*, writes about different kinds of crowds, and cites as one of the most frightening the "baiting crowd": "This concentration on killing is of a special kind and of an unsurpassed intensity. Everyone wants to participate," Canetti wrote. "If he cannot hit him himself he wants to see others hit him.... Every arm is thrust out as if they all belonged to one and the same creature.... There is no risk because the crowd has immense superiority on their side."

In 1994, a high ranking NIH geneticist who was also a friend of Duesberg's, Dr. Stephen O'Brien, called Duesberg and said he urgently needed to see him about a professional matter. He flew in from Bethesda the next day and the two attended the opera in San Francisco together, before settling down to talk. Duesberg was hopeful that O'Brien came bearing good news, that maybe he would be considered for an NIH grant again. "I said OK, what is my big surprise?" Duesberg recalls. "'Will I get a grant again?' This was very high on my mind at the time."

Instead, O'Brien pulled a manuscript from the inside pocket of his jacket. Headlined, "HIV Causes AIDS: Koch's Postulates Fulfilled," it had three names at the bottom: Stephen O'Brien, Robert Gallo, and Peter Duesberg.

Remarkably, the essay had been commissioned by *Nature's* John Maddox. If Duesberg would only sign, O'Brien implored, he could have everything back, be back at the top again, back in "the club." O'Brien told Duesberg that if he signed it, the paper would be on the presses by the following Tuesday—that he would fly to London immediately and deliver it to Maddox.

Unfailingly polite, Duesberg and his wife, Siggi Sachs, drove his old friend to the airport and said he would give the matter careful consideration. He already knew what he was going to do.

He sent the manuscript back to London the next day, but this time it was two papers. One, the original, with his own name removed, and a second paper which consisted of his rebuttal. Neither was published, and Duesberg hasn't been published in *Nature* in the years since.

I asked Duesberg whether O'Brien actually spelled out that the signing of the paper would reverse his fortune.

"Yeah, of course," he said. "He said I would be accepted again.... That I had done such good work on cancer and onco- genes and they all respected me for that, but in the case of AIDS I was out of my depths. There I had made, unfortunately, a trag- ic misjudgment which could be corrected now. I would be back in the lap of the establishment, back in my deserved position. This is how he said it."

Not wanting to embarrass his old colleague, Duesberg withheld O'Brien's identity when he published detailed accounts of the AIDS controversy in his book *Inventing the AIDS Virus* in 1996. But he revealed O'Brien's identity in the Italian edition of the book after O'Brien's name appeared on two anti-Duesberg pieces claim- ing Koch's postulates had been fulfilled and HIV was the cause of AIDS. These claims were cited in the "Durban Declaration," a peti- tion signed by 5,000 scientists, insisting that there is no question whatsoever that HIV causes AIDS, a declaration that was published in *Nature,* and in the *New York Times,* on the eve of the International Conference on AIDS in Durban in 2002.

Referring to O'Brien, Duesberg said: "So I didn't spare his name anymore after he published these articles and I realized that he is a hardcore NIH activist...or whatever it is...NIH *scientist.* By this I mean hard-line NIH scientist whose opinion is predeter- mined by the institution...like the HIV/AIDS website of the NIH, where these miserable correlations are cited as proof that

HIV is causing AIDS and meets Koch's Postulates! Science by the declaration of 5,000 scientists including Nobel Prize winners!"

"It reminds me of the one story I know about Einstein. You know Einstein was told after he left Germany that hundreds of German physicists had signed a declaration that his relatively was 'questionable' and 'dubious.' It was considered 'Jewish science.' Anyway, his answer was: Why so many? It only takes one if you have proof. That was Einstein's answer. And in a way that was my reaction also. It's intimidating, of course, if you hear this. Five thousand scientists signing a petition that this is the cause of AIDS, including Nobel Prize winners.... "

"They took him out—just took him right out." says Richard Strohman, a retired UC Berkeley emeritus professor of cell biology, best known for his important work on muscle, and recently for his widely read critiques of the extravagant claims made for the medical benefits that will come from the completion of the sequencing of the human genome.

"The system works," says David Rasnick. "It's as good as a bullet to the head."

I asked her if we could talk about Peter Duesberg and she nodded, and walked me down the corridor into her office. She asked that I not identify her, and that I say only that she has known him for "a considerable time," and that she is a UC Berkeley scientist.

"I am not fond of this topic," she said, as I sat down in the chair opposite her, and explained what I was there to examine: Peter Duesberg's potential rehabilitation. The scientist knew Duesberg well, as did her husband, who apparently was "furious" at him when he, in her words, "disgraced" himself with the HIV debate.

"I don't think Peter is necessarily wrong," she said. "But he had a fatal flaw. He went public. I think he hurt himself. He didn't understand the real world."

"Peter doesn't have a bad bone in his body, but he's childish. I think he sees the world in bright colors."

"Bright colors?" I said.

"Yes. He did it to himself, you know. Everything that's happened. You see, he wouldn't give up an idea. He went at it with a hammer. He may well be 3,000 percent right, but he upset an awful lot of people through his doggedness, which only made him more dogged."

"So that's not a value, then, in science...being dogged?" I asked.

"He's been unpopular his entire career. You can't help but love him. He's here because nobody will have him.... Nobody believed in him because what he was doing was overturning generally held views. They felt betrayed."

"They felt betrayed?"

"Yes, they felt attacked." She paused. "Let me explain something. Political savvy is intrinsic to a scientific career. You don't just stand up and say that everybody is wrong."

"What should he have done though, given that he did think they were wrong?"

She shook her head and smiled. "There's no such thing as totally right or totally wrong."

"In *science*? There's no such thing as totally right or totally wrong?"

She waved her hand, as though we were talking about something faintly banal. "Listen, it's passé now. He would have been OK if he had just done things as convention dictates.... I wouldn't want his life. In the department, they'd laugh and talk about him. He was very irritating to the department. He carried his ideas too far.... If he had just *apologized*, he would have been resurrected long ago," she said.

"But how could he apologize unless he felt he had done something wrong?" I asked.

"Peter may be right about HIV," she said. "But there's an industry now.... I don't think Peter understands what's going on. He thinks everybody should be friendly. Maybe that's it. He's like a child, he really is."

Before I left she wanted to stress one more time that Peter Duesberg had brought all his miseries and punishments onto himself, that there was no "conspiracy," something I heard repeated by several others on the anti-Duesberg side of the fence.

I asked her if I could feel free to quote her and she adamantly said she did not want to be identified. We negotiated about what I could say about her, and wound up with only the most elliptical identification. She feared "they" would figure out who she was. As I was leaving she said, "I don't want to go on record saying anything for *or* against Peter."

Today's scientists are wholly dependent for their survival upon the will of a conjoined financial megalopolis connecting government, academia, and the bio-tech and pharmaceutical industries. If you talk to them, they almost all speak of fear—fear of losing their funding. Minds attuned, consciously and unconsciously, to the roar of the industry, scientists writing grants that are designed to feed and fuel it—writing more and more grants in shorter and shorter intervals than ever before.

"You have to write a grant a year almost," says Richard Strohman. "And you have to write four to get one, if you're any good. I got out just in time. Everybody who's still in there says the same thing. It's going to hell in a hand basket. Before the bio-tech boom, we never had this incessant urging to produce something useful, meaning profitable. Under these circumstances, everybody is caught up in it. Grants, millions of dollars flowing into laboratories, careers and stars being made. The only way to be a successful scientist today is to follow consensus. The academy has become the technology it invented. It's lost its scientific edge and replaced it with a technology that follows the market. The tension between the two is that science is primarily a generator of surprises, whereas technology is anything but surprises. If you're going to produce something and put it on the market, you don't want any goddamn surprises. You've got the next quarter to report and you don't want any bad news. It's all about the short term now.

"Fifty, sixty years ago there was still a pluralism in the life sciences. I used to be the chairman of the zoology department at Berkeley. It's gone now. I call this the intellectual urban renewal program. They tore down the neighborhoods and put up all these high-rises and nobody talks to one another."

The myth of science is that it is a profession that prizes curiosity, confusion, and wonder. You think of science and you think of Gregor Mendel poking around in his pea garden in Brno, or Darwin studying his fossils in the candle-lit cabin of the HMS *Beagle*.

Alexander Fleming with his moldering Petri dishes would not exist today. The mold that became penicillin wouldn't grow, because the window in the lab wouldn't be open.

Peter Duesberg is alone, at his favorite outdoor table of the UC Berkeley coffee house, La Strada, typing on his laptop. At 66, he is a slender man, average height, with white, wavy hair that doesn't do anything crazy. Professorial hair. Blue eyes that have been described as having a twinkle and a German face that you could call boyish. He's wearing a white shirt and a navy knit vest, and he's typing, with an empty cappuccino cup next to him and a plate with crumbs that he dusts off his fingertips.

The café is noisy, students, adorned with the body-décor of would-be rebellion—piercings, tattoos, torn clothes—stream past and take no notice of him.

A man comes over, a student of about forty-five, just as I sit down, and greets Duesberg warmly. The man, who thinks Duesberg is correct about HIV and AIDS, says: "I have friends hereon campus who think 9/11 was an inside job. But your stuff..." He shakes his head and laughs. "It's too radical for them. They refuse to even talk about it."

I contacted the Berkeley deans who oppose Duesberg and asked if they would speak to me. None of them agreed to an interview. Some didn't reply and others said they were leaving on vacations. One of them, Professor Michael Botchan, replied via email with this: "Conspiracies in the academy don't exist as they did in Galileo's time—really. Now, Peter Duesberg has a theory that aneuploidy is necessary *and* sufficient for all cancers. If he is having trouble getting funded over an extensive period of time, it means that his peers really don't think much of his notions. Any other slant would in my opinion be way off the mark."

David Steele, Duesberg's attorney hands me a large black folder of correspondences between Duesberg and the Berkeley administration. "Read it for yourself," he says. "They are egregiously biased and take shots at him at every turn. The ethic among these guys is if you have a chance to take a whack at Duesberg, you never miss that chance. It's a whole culture. They reward each other for it."

At least twice, his request for a merit pay increase has had to go to a new reviewer, as mediators have found them to be biased in their assessment of Duesberg's work, but it is difficult if not impossible to find an impartial reviewer in the Department of Molecular and Cell Biology at Berkeley. Reviewing the dossier, one exchange in particular caught my attention. It was a simple thing: Duesberg had written to a secretary asking about the teaching schedule for the upcoming semester. Surprisingly, the reply came from Duesberg's colleague, Stuart Linn, who wrote: "Surely, Peter, as a member of the NAS [National Academy of Sciences], you can look up the lab days and divide them by 3. In the event that you cannot, there are 44 days of class and an exam at the end of each (unless you want to have the exam at the beginning, or don't want to have one), leaving 41 days of lab."

Linn went on at length to list the exams, and concluded: "If this doesn't work for you, you are free to give lectures on AIDS, not give an exam, etc., but don't ask Sharon Lindley to worry about it, as it is not her responsibility."

This was one rare instance where Duesberg showed emotion. "Surely, Stuart," he wrote to his colleague, "Why would you have to address me as a member of the NAS in criticizing me for not knowing when exactly my section of MCB 11OL starts next February? I can not help it that I was elected into the NAS—but, I also can not help it that you were not."

During 2004 and 2005, a scientific article and several commentaries appeared in *Nature Genetics*, *Science*, and *Nature* that represented a shift of focus onto aneuploidy as the "casual link" in cancer. The abstract of the article, which generated a fusillade of praise, concluded: "These data strongly support a casual link between aneuploidy and cancer development." The paper kept gene mutations in the picture, but moved them to the background and aneuploidy to the foreground. Neither the article itself nor any of the commentaries took more than passing note of Duesberg's tireless efforts in giving aneuploidy its new luster.

Duesberg has not, however, been completely airbrushed out of the picture, having received word from the editors at *Science* that they would be publishing a letter raising a few of the problems associated with attributing to aneuploidy the essentials of cancer cell initiation and yet still insisting that this massive genetic change is brought about by mutations in specific genes. The letter also calls understated attention to the fact that Duesberg has published extensively on the importance of aneuploidy in the evolution of the cancer cell. "In view of these problems, my colleagues and I have proposed that carcinogenesis is initiated by a random aneuploidy, which is generated either by a carcinogen or spontaneously," it says.

"The flag they're running up the pole now is like aneuploidy flanked by mutations," says George Miklos, commenting on the latest aneuploidy renaissance. "What it does is it gets them out of the old bind, and allows them to transition out of mutations and oncogenes and tumor suppressors, so that eventually people won't think about all that anymore. Biologists are hypothesis hoarders, they never throw anything away. Unlike in physics where data are clean and if things aren't right the hypothesis falls—biologists never come out and say they were wrong. Ever. But this is a clear transition away from the old dogma."

On a bright winter morning in early December 2005, my friend Rob Drescher and I took a cab up to Mt. Sinai Medical Center in New York City to hear Peter Duesberg give a talk about aneuploidy.

Every seat was filled and there were people sitting and crouching in every square inch of floor space. Most were students, some were older professors, and scientists with white coats—but mostly students. I found a small space near the door and crouched down. Duesberg was saying: "This is speciation, not mutation. Forty-six is what we try to keep together to look like Robert Wainberg or George Bush, but sometimes it falls apart." The audience roared with laughter. This was a room filled with people who would catch a reference to Duesberg's dispute with Dr. Wainberg. "If confirmed," Duesberg said, "the chromosomal theory would have revealed the first Achilles heel we have yet to see in cancer—pre-neoplastic aneuploidy, which can be detected ctyogenetically, in routine biopsies, pap smears, etc., and this offers new chances for cancer treatment."

He described coming to America in the 1960s, "when we all thought cancer was caused by viruses. We were one family. Because retroviruses don't kill cells, we figured here we have potential cancer viruses...but unfortunately there was in the end no evidence that viruses cause cancer...."

I wrote down the phrase "retroviruses don't kill cells." There was no protest when he said it. This was a room of America's next generation of cancer researchers. Was it because they did not deal with AIDS that they accepted this truth as self-evident? If retroviruses, as a class, are universally known *not to kill cells*, then how could that one—HIV—do something no other virus in its class could do?

After he finished, many of the students asked versions of the same question: Is it possible you are wrong, that it's the other way around, that genetic mutations cause aneuploidy which in turn causes cancer? He explained why this was unfortunately not possible.

I stepped out of the room to have a word with one of the cancer researchers who had organized the talk, Dr. Lu Wang. I asked him what Peter Duesberg's reputation is, today, in the field of cancer. "He is still very respected in the oncogene field," he said. Nodding toward the window he continued: "The room is jammed. He has made a good argument. We all have to go home and think about it."

I asked him to elaborate on whether Duesberg's current theory on cancer and aneuploidy is, as some say, "part of the answer," or perhaps more than that.

"I think he is an experimental genius," he said. "If he wants to perform experiments, he should be able to."

I noted how bright the students' faces were, how curious. On the other hand, one could sense their conflict—a sense of obligation to "nail him," as though to pay a debt to their own teachers, or hold on to the past before they board the train to the future. How can they get on that train if Duesberg is driving it? Who would they be betraying?

Later, my friend said I had missed the part where the students had asked Duesberg how many lab assistants he had. It was a question that really asked: "If I follow you, do you have anything to offer in terms of worldly comforts?"

The day after the lecture at Mt. Sinai, Duesberg called and said he had a bit of free time and asked if I wanted to have a cup of coffee. I met him in the lobby of his upper east side hotel, where I found him at the concierge desk asking the girl there, who was from Bosnia, questions about her life. The walls were bursting with lush Christmas décor, and the floors were sparkling marble.

We chose a café, and we ordered some tea and sandwiches. For some inexplicable reason, the waiter seemed furious at

Duesberg. He kept slamming down his plates and addressing him as though he were some kind of bum—as though he had violated a serious but unknown code. When it came time to leave, Duesberg paid the bill, and I started fiddling with bills for a tip, assuming we might leave a paltry one.

"Why don't we make a really clear statement instead?" said Duesberg. He cleared the table of *all* money, and we left.

Back in California, Duesberg invited me to his home, a modest, comfortable affair. Duesberg and his wife Siggi Sachs, an attractive German woman with a throaty laugh, are setting the table for a small dinner party, and arguing about the cheese platter. Duesberg sprinkles coarse salt on a whole grilled salmon, and says something in German to an elderly woman seated at the end of the table—a colleague who housed him and his family in Mannheim all those years when he went back to work on aneuploidy. Also present is a close friend of the couple, a sixty-five-year-old librarian named Fred Cline, who, ironically, is a gay man—and I say ironically only because the common accusation is that Duesberg is a homophobe.

"Homophobe? I don't think so. I've been in a hot tub with Peter," says Cline and laughs.

Siggi and Peter Duesberg have an eight-year-old son named Max, who speaks German and English, and Duesberg has three grown daughters from a previous marriage.

"I can't even go to the campus. The hostility just pours out from every corner," says Siggi. She puts down a plate of cheese on the table and says, insistently: "Science has become such a rotten thing. Lots of mediocre people who don't want to risk anything. *They're egomaniacs.*"

She spoke of the social ostracization the family suffers. "We are never invited anywhere. Never. It's very hard and I'm so tired of it. The AIDS thing *that* they will never give up, they will fight it to the end."

Max climbs into his father's lap, and Duesberg whispers something to him and they laugh. I ask Max if he wants to be a scientist when he grows up. "I want to be that last," he says. "In the last part of my life."

We get to talking about the 1989 earthquake, the big one. "Were you here?" I ask Duesberg.

"I was here, yes," he says distractedly.

"Peter was in the *lab*," Siggi insists, with a combination of annoyance and affection. "Harry Rubin came running in and said, 'Peter we have to get out of here it's an earthquake!'" She laughs. "And you know Peter, you know how he is. *He wouldn't leave.* He said, 'I'm finishing my experiment.'"

SATURDAY, JUNE 11, 1988. STOCKHOLM, SWEDEN.
Two subway stops from central Stockholm, amid patches of lush
forest and grassy hills, stands a monstrous, bright orange structure
of cement and glass. Inside, the atmosphere is sterile and futuristic,
with uniformed guards carrying metal detectors, computers hanging from ceilings flashing messages, and carpeted glass tunnels
connecting the vast halls. A large black screen in the main
entrance says, "Welcome to the Fourth International Conference
on AIDS. Stockholm International Fairs, June 12-16, 1988.
The time is 1:03 p.m."

The weather in Stockholm is perfect. Conference delegates mill
around the Old City in Stockholm, awed by its flawless charm,
shopping for Kosta Boda crystal, Marabou chocolate, and clogs, in
the hours between registration and the opening ceremony.

The tidy blond woman behind the counter smiles, hands me my
badge and the two catalogues of abstracts, each as thick as the
Manhattan Yellow Pages and twice as heavy. "Relax, dear dele-
gate," one of them begins. "You have 2,000 valuable minutes in
which to meet more than 6,000 other delegates and to digest
more than 3,000 scientific communications. Relax in the awareness that it is not only impossible, but hardly worthwhile, to try
to comprehend the entire conference."

In one of the two main poster halls, a few dozen people have
already started setting up booths and tacking up posters. The first
familiar face I see is Bob Kunst from Cure AIDS Now (CAN),

whose booth is already set up with flyers, buttons, and petitions. The last time I saw him was at last year's AIDS conference in Washington, DC. "How are you?" I ask. "Fed up," he says. "My best friend died last week. Since the last time I saw you, I've been to over forty funerals."

SUNDAY, JUNE 12.

Dr. Robert Gallo's voice booms out over the public address system. "The period of 1982-1984 saw dramatic advances in research. We were able to prove that HIV was the cause of the disease; the virus was reproduced in mass, continuous tissue culture; and blood tests were developed that saved thousands of lives by preventing the spread of the virus. The antiviral program that followed, based on findings about HIV, led to the development of AZT. It has been said that this is the most incredible advance in a new disease in the history of biomedical science."

The introductory ceremony has been going on for two hours now and the man seated to my left is fast asleep, lulled by the droning, hollow rhetoric of the speakers, all of them extolling the incredible feats of science. Beginning with the prime minister of Sweden and ending with Bob Gallo, each speaker repeats the claims as if they were political slogans:

"Never before in the history of disease has science advanced so rapidly. In only four years, since we discovered the virus, we have been able to..."

"We know more about HIV than any other virus in the history of science...."

And so on.

Both Gallo and Luc Montagnier, "co-discovers of HIV," centered their speeches on defending the theory that HIV is the cause of AIDS, which had been strongly challenged during the past year. Montagnier said that the evidence is overwhelming that HIV-1 and -2 are the agents, because HIV-2 has now caused AIDS in macaque monkeys. He talked about Simian Immunodeficiency Viruses (SIV) causing SAIDS in rhesus monekeys, Feline Immunodeficiency Virus (FIV) causing Feline AIDS (FAIDS), African Green Monkeys, Lentiviruses, and mutations of HIV. The most alarming point he made was that people who are testing negative for HIV may have "hidden" infections, which would explain why so many people with AIDS test negative for HIV antibodies.

Gallo offered a long list of reason to believe that HIV is the cause of AIDS, yet concluded, oddly enough, by introducing a new herpes virus, HBLV or HHV-6, which he said is "definitely a co-factor in the development of AIDS."

Back in the press room, typewriters are clicking frantically. Two Canadian reporters are trying to straighten it all out.

"Did you understand any of that?" one of them wonders.

"Well, yeah. HIV is the primary cause of AIDS, but there are several other viruses that act as co-factors—like HHV-6 or whatever, and HIV-2."

"But why is HIV-2 the one that makes monkeys sick?" asked the reporter, trying to clarify the labyrinthian differences between HIV-1, SIV, and HIV-2. HIV-2, first discovered two years after HIV-1, is commonly understood to be more prevalent in Africa and less pathogenic than HIV-2; it is also believed to be more difficult to spread, even though it is widely believed that AIDS transmission in Africa is much higher than in the West.

I spot Randy Shilts, the *San Francisco Chronicle* reporter who was catapulted to fame with his book *And the Band Played On*, a piercing exposé of the corrupt and bungling politics of AIDS in the United States. I introduce myself.

Shilts tells me that a group of people are going around the conference, targeting gay people in particular and trying to convince them that Gallo's not such a bad guy after all.

"They said to me," recalls Shilts, rolling his eyes in disgust, "'Do you know that Dr. Gallo was going to leave science because of your book? Why can't you write about all the good things he's doing?' 'I'd be very surprised if Dr. Gallo left science,' I told them. 'How else is he going to get 7,000 people in a room to get up and cheer for him?'"

MONDAY, JUNE 13.

In one of the two main poster halls, all the scientific abstracts are tacked up on big white boards. After an hour of walking around trying desperately to take in and understand their meaning, I feel dizzy and confused, blinded by science. '3' AZIDOTHYMA-DINE (AZT) PREVENTS THE DISSEMINATION OF RETROVIRUS IN LP-BM5 MuLV INFECTED C57BL/6 MICE. I may as well be trying to understand Chinese. Two major facts do emerge, though, almost immediately: 1) That an overwhelming majority of the antiviral therapy abstracts are on AZT, the only drug that has received FDA approval as an AIDS therapy. 2) That most of the abstracts on AZT conclude, in one way or another, that AZT, although it is toxic, is effective against AIDS.

The most disturbing thing I hear about AZT at the entire conference comes from Sam Broder, the man behind AZT from the National Cancer Institute, who says that we should start giving AZT to HIV-positive asymptomatic women, so that their unborn children can absorb it through the placenta and better their chances of never developing AIDS.

The most important abstract of the conference, however, seemed to be #2662. An army researcher, Dr. Shyh-Ching Lo, from the Armed Forces Institute of Pathology, isolated an agent from an AIDS patient that causes AIDS symptoms and death in animals. And it isn't HIV.

The authors of the abstracts are at their posters between 11:00 and 12:00 every day. Dr. Lo is alone in front of his poster. When he spots the PRESS on my badge, he is cautious, saying "I don't want to get involved in all the political conflicts; I've been burned a few times and I want to make sure the science isn't sacrificed."

Assuring him that I just want to know about his abstracts, I asked him if he really isolated a virus from an AIDS patient that is totally different from HIV.

"Yes," he says, "we're not even so sure it's a virus. Let's just call it an agent. We know it's contagious and we know it's DNA contained, which is a difference from the retrovirus HIV. The agent does not contain any reverse transcriptase activity, which is the hallmark for a retrovirus, so we know we're not dealing with a retrovirus. If it is a virus at all, it is a DNA virus. We injected this agent in four monkeys and in seven-nine months they all died."

"And what kind of symptoms did they have?"

"Mainly weight loss, not associated with significant diarrhea. In the terminal stage, they have very low white blood cell counts, and they also had very persistent fever in the earlier course of the disease."

"Do you believe that this agent has anything to do with the etiology of AIDS or the development of AIDS in a person, or is this just another opportunistic agent?"

"Obviously, any AIDS patient is immunocompromised and has a much higher chance of getting opportunistic infections. Right now we don't know if this is an opportunistic infection or if it has a significant role in the etiology of AIDS."

"Do you think it has any relationship to Dr. Gallo's HBLV or HHV-6?"

"No. Genetic analysis has been done to compare it with HBLV and we're quite confident that it's not the same virus."

A man who has been standing nearby, listening attentively to our conversation, introduces himself. He is a former employee of the New York City Department of Health, who resigned because of the AIDS program. He's very interested in Lo's agent. I ask him why.

"Well," he says, "when someone says they've found an new infectious particle in an AIDS patient, one immediately wonders if it has anything to do with the development of AIDS. Maybe HIV and this virus work together. Since it's a DNA virus, it may be easier to treat it. We are able to treat herpes, for example. If this is true, it's extremely significant because it means we might have another route to a therapy for AIDS. It is a very, very fascinating finding. I think it's the most important abstract at the whole conference."

"What do you think," I ask him, "about Gallo's HBLV?"

"I haven't had time assess it, really. I think Dr Gallo wants us to believe in a certain religion, and that religion is H-I-V. He wants that to be the cause of AIDS and he want to get a Nobel Prize. Even if he finds another virus, he doesn't want to change the thinking right now."

Bob Gallo is standing in the middle of the main hall, deep in conversation. His manner is rushed, intense, with sudden gestures and a blunt delivery. Wanting to speak to him about Lo's virus and HBLV, I hover in his general area for about thirty minutes, hoping he'll finish his conversation. While I am standing there, a man walks up to me, hands me his camera, and ask if I would take a picture of him and Dr. Gallo.

"In Egypt, we like Dr. Gallo very much," he says. "More than we like Dr. Montagnier." I imagine Egyptian TV reporters stopping people at the marketplace in Cairo and asking them who their favorite discoverer is: Gallo or Montagnier? He walks up to Gallo, shakes his hand, they both smile, and I take the picture.

Handing back the camera, I say, "Hello, Dr. Gallo. May I ask you a few questions?"

"I don't have time right now. I was on my way out," he snaps. "Where's Flossy? Flossy, come on! We're late." Gallo strides over to Flossy Wong Staal, his coworker and closest companion, followed by a team of TV reporters. "Here he is," Staal announces proudly, "the famous Dr. Gallo." The reporters flock to him, literally jabbing each other to get closer. They start making their way toward the exit.

"Are we going to get a vaccine soon, Dr. Gallo?" asks one Swedish reporter.

"Well," says Gallo, "the basic science is progressing extremely rapidly and very well. But the hardest thing is still left to do—to get rid of the disease, right? I think it's do-able, and that's a sincere statement. I think it will be solved, not thanks to public education, but thanks to science. But I'm not going to tell you when."

He bolts through the revolving doors. I missed him. I go to the press room and put in a request to interview him, fully aware that it will never happen. I'm told Dr. Gallo will be holding a closed, very exclusive press conference tomorrow, and that I'd be wasting my time trying to get in.

"I promise not to ask him anything," I plead. The press officer laughs.

TUESDAY, JUNE 14.

On my way to the main poster hall, I see Dr. Anthony Fauci, the head of the National Institute of Allergies and Infectious Diseases

(NIAID), walking towards the cafeteria. "Excuse me, Dr. Fauci," I say. "I'm confused by Dr. Gallo's speech. How important is HBLV in the development of AIDS? How can he say that it's 'definitely a cofactor in the development of AIDS,' yet all we test for and worry about is HIV?"

"I think," says Fauci, "the point he was probably making is that it very well may serve as a co-factor, an inducing factor. He wasn't talking about anything primary. It's very clear that the primary etiologic agent is unquestionably HIV-1."

"But isn't the problem with HIV that it doesn't kill T-cells?"

"No...well, it does, actually. That's the point that again gets confused. If you look at HIV in the test tube, it kills T-cells very efficiently. The thing in the body is that it does it in a very gradual way. But you can definitely, unequivocally demonstrate that HIV does kill T-4 cells."

"So a co-factor isn't entirely necessary, then, but if there is a co-factor, HBLV is being considered?"

"Exactly," smiles Fauci.

Jim Fouratt, from the PWA (People With AIDS) health group in New York City, walks up from behind and grabs my arm. "Come on," he says, pulling me toward the plenary halls, "the guy who injected himself is speaking at two."

"Who?" I ask, jogging to keep up with him.

"Zagury or whatever his name is. He's trying to develop a vaccine and he's used himself as a model." We run into Randy Shilts, who is headed in the opposite direction. "Randy, come on," shouts Jim. "You've got to come hear Zagury." Shilts follows us. We find the workshop, titled "Vaccine Development and Planning for Trials," and are ushered in. The room is absolutely packed. It's hot and there is no oxygen. We prop up against the wall and strain to hear the French scientist's words.

Daniel Zagury may be the only scientist at the conference who, in the course of his research, has put his life on the line. Zagury injected himself with HIV antibody particles in order to devlop HIV antibodies, which he hopes may evolve into a vaccine. After his presentation he was mobbed by reporters. When asked how his health was, he replied, "I've never felt better."

The bottom line about a vaccine against AIDS was delivered by Nobel prize winner David Baltimore, who said, "This conference will not reveal any good news about vaccines or treatments. There are many hypotheses, but few solid advances."

Some experts at the conference went so far as to say that the very idea of developing a vaccine is fruitless—impossible. Every attempt to vaccinate monkeys and apes against HIV has failed. If it were a simple matter of creating antibodies, we would have had a vaccine long ago, because the body does this naturally. In fact, when we refer to somebody "having the AIDS virus," we actual-ly mean they have antibodies to it. If natural antibodies do not provide immunity, why should vaccine induced antibodies miraculously do so?

WEDNESDAY, JUNE 15.

The very first thing you see when you enter the main exhibition hall is a huge white banner with blue letters that says "WELL-COME." Burroughs-Wellcome, the company that owns AZT, has an enclosed area as big as two large living rooms, with wall-to-wall carpeting and plush sofas in matching ash grey. Sixteen large video screens cover one wall. The images on the screens, synchronized to a cheap, instrumental disco song, alternate between scientists holding up test tubes in laboratories, pills being funneled into bottles zipping on a conveyor belt, and masses of people, in slow motion, crossing a street ("The virus is spreading throughout the population...."). Huge glass windows, posters, and banners bear the Wellcome emblem, an illuminated blue unicorn, standing on the hollow slogan: "Wellcome...Meeting the Viral Challenge."

Every other time the video runs, the music stops and a British accent narrates, "In 1984, three years after the first cases of AIDS were reported, a retrovirus was identified as the causative agent.... Since the fifties, the Wellcome Foundation has been doing extensive antiviral research, and so it was natural for Wellcome to be at the forefront of the effort to find an effective therapy for AIDS. In November 1984, just months after HIV had been identified, scientists at the U.S. research laboratories of the Wellcome Foundation Limited screened a Thymadine analogue. This agent showed activity against the HIV virus.... Today AZT is our only hope against the dreaded disease. Thousands of patients around the world are..."

"You've got to be kidding," I say under my breath.

"Pardon?" A young man in a grey suit and Burroughs-Wellcome badge looks at me indignantly."

"Your video doesn't mention certain details about AZT," I say flatly, "like that it costs $10,000 per year to take, or that it was a cancer drug seventeen years ago but was considered too toxic for people to be subjected to. Or that 50 percent of all AIDS patients can't take it because...

"Never mind." I keep walking on through the huge poster hall, half expecting to hear Orwell's haunting chant: WAR IS PEACE, FREEDOM IS SLAVERY, IGNORANCE IS STRENGTH.

I am standing on line at one of the cafeterias, where shrimp sandwiches are almost ten dollars each, and I overhear two men in front of me discussing the latest rumor: that AZT stocks have dropped twenty points since Gallo's speech about HBLV, because it is feared that HIV may not cause AIDS after all. I go back to the Wellcome camp and ask the man in the grey suit if the rumor is true. He says he knows nothing about it.

The only expression of Swedish gays fighting AIDS came from a booth bannered "RFSL" (Riksforbundet for Sexual Liberation). Two bearded gay men are sitting behind the booth, wearing ACT UP (AIDS Coalition to Unleash Power) stickers with the motto "Silence=Death" on their badges. There are two bowls on the counter, one with potato chips, one with condoms. Next to the condoms is a stack of invitations to tomorrow night's "Jack-Off Party" in the old town. The cover of the invitation has a vague drawing of four naked men standing in a circle holding their hands on each other's buttocks. I open it and read:

Rules:
*Street clothes, including pants or shorts, MUST be removed upon entering. Nudity, save footwear, is encouraged.
*Activity is STRICTLY J/O: Solo, by the score, in a huddle, across the room, stroke, rub, pull, exhibit, touch, hold.
*There will be NO ass play OR activities that result in any exchange of body fluid (semen, urine, saliva).
Relax and enjoy
We are friendly as well as horny
Doors open 8-9
Snacks and Non-Alcoholic Beverages

The two guys in the booth looked bored. Sweden currently has so far had 192 AIDS cases, of whom eighty-nine have died. So far, out of a population of 8.4 million, 1,816 are reported HIV-positive. Of every country in the world, Sweden is the country that has carried out the greatest number of HIV tests per inhabitant. But the most startling news about AIDS in Sweden is this: Sweden is the only country that has a law allowing compulsory isolation for HIV-infected people. The government has selected an island in Stockholm's archipelago as the quarantine sight for any HIV-infected person who does not abide by his or her doctor's sexual-behavior regulations.

I ask the two guys in the RFSL booth about this. They tell me that four people have been sentenced to isolation on the island so far. "It's crazy," says one of them. "Doctors can say anything they want, and who can prove it's true?"

"HIV-positive people can be locked up in total isolation on the basis of pure hearsay, of arbitrary speculation about an individual being a contamination threat to his or her fellow human beings. No proof whatsoever is required," says Hasse Ytterberg, President of the National Swedish Federation for Gay and Lesbian Rights, in a speech at the Candlelight March held during the conference. "The Swedish AIDS legislation is probably one of the most repressive in the world."

The Swedish press's approach to AIDS is terror-oriented, making no distinction between HIV-antibody positive status and AIDS. *Aftonbladet*, the leading evening newspaper, ran a cover story on the first day of the conference about the plight of HIV-positive children in Sweden, and the only themes presented were death, despair, shock, terminal illness, and isolation. This bothered me. Living in New York City, I'd grown accustomed to seeing people with AIDS fight like hell to stay alive.

"Are you guys connected to the gay communities in New York and LA?" I ask the men in the RFSL booth. "Do the people with AIDS in Sweden know there are new, effective therapies that offer a better chance of survival than AZT? Do they know that there are long-term survivors of AIDS, or that being HIV-positive is not the same as being dead?"

The two men give me blank stares. "Yes, we know about all that," one of them says meekly.

"Then why aren't you talking about it? I mean, you are the only ones who can reach people...people with AIDS. You have to encourage them to fight. Try to get some articles published in the papers or something."

"Yes, I hear what you are saying," one of them says coldly, "but it's not as easy as you think. This is not the United States, this is Sweden. And most people are so terrified of letting it be known that they have HIV or AIDS that they'd rather keep a low profile. They'd rather be quiet."

"Show them your stickers," I say. "Silence=Death. There's nothing to be afraid of if you're dead, is there?"

They start to look irritated now. In the neighboring booth, a video about a girl who finds out she is HIV-positive is playing. She's sitting in her doctor's office. She gets the test results and starts crying and screaming frantically. "Why me!? Why the fuck should I get this? I've been clean for two years now!" Her doctor just sits there and finally he says, in a very placid, parental tone, "Eva...I'm very sorry. I really am, but the most important thing right now is that you tell me who you've been with so we can warn them."

"Like that!" I say. "What good does a video like that do? They don't even know for sure if HIV is the real cause of AIDS, so why is her doctor treating her like she's already dead? That's the kind of thing I'm talking about."

"What are you talking about? Of course HIV is the cause of AIDS. How can you say it's not?"

"I didn't say it's not," I say as calmly as I can. "I just said they're not 100 percent certain anymore. Even Gallo himself said that HBLV is a definite co-factor in the development of AIDS, so that must mean that HIV alone may not cause AIDS."

A Swedish social worker joins the conversation. I tell him about Duesberg's theory that HIV isn't the cause of AIDS. Within five minutes he's screaming at the top of his lungs, his face bright red, his index finger jabbing my shoulder.

"YOU'RE JUST TRYING TO DENY REALITY! EVERY SINGLE PERSON WHO GETS HIV IS GOING TO DIE. MAYBE NOT TODAY OR TOMORROW, BUT EVENTUALLY."

Another Swede, a researcher, joins in, "You're the one who's denying reality," he says to the social worker. "If you knew anything about the mechanisms of HIV, you would be skeptical of it too. You're not being objective."

"I AM BEING OBJECTIVE. ARE YOU SUGGESTING THAT PEOPLE DON'T USE CONDOMS? IS THAT WHAT YOU WANT?"

"No, of course not…"

Jim walks up and pulls me gently away from them, saying he has somebody he wants to meet. "I should have told you," he says. "Whatever you do, don't mention Duesberg here. Just don't mention him. I brought him up at a press conference yesterday, and this crazy Swedish woman followed me around for a half hour, yelling at me."

Jim takes off and I keep walking. This particular stretch of the conference is focused on AIDS prevention and education. There are condoms in every color and instructions on how to use them in every language. Video screens are everywhere, with naked

couples, heterosexual and homosexual, caressing each other while
somber narrators talk about the HIV threat and how to have safer
sex. "Bleachman," the AIDS-prevention superhero created by the
San Francisco AIDS Foundation, is standing in full costume,
dressed as a jug of bleach, handing out leaflets about cleaning
needles, and two Danish junkies have a poster exhibition that says
that it's not being a junkie that gives you AIDS—it's dirty needles.
The posters explain how you can keep shooting drugs, as long as
you clean your works.

Back in the pressroom, reporters are trying very hard not to panic.
"Does anybody know what's really going on here?" I ask the
woman from *Le Monde* at the next typewriter. "No, not really,"
she says, "but you're not supposed to at conferences like this.
How could you?"

I remember what the chairman of the conference, Lars Olof
Kallings, said in his introductory speech. "A scientific conference
can be looked upon as a mosaic, in this case with more than 3,000
pieces. Each piece, however well-shaped and beautiful, does
not tell us very much. But when the pieces are put together a
picture develops. . . ."

THURSDAY, JUNE 16.

Mathilde Krim, Chairman of AmFAR, the American Foundation
for AIDS Research, is sitting at a small table in the AmFAR
booth. I ask her how she feels about the conference.

"I feel that on the scientific front, they're going for a period of
consolidation. For the first time in the history of this epidemic,
we know what we're dealing with, and there are solid foundations
built to address the problem. For the first time, I think, we're
seeing AIDS the right way."

"More so than at the last conference?" I ask.

"Yes, much more so. The Washington meeting was very divided. There was a kind of anger in the air that was very destructive. It was against government inaction. Every public official who appeared at that conference was booed. That mood is gone today. I don't see that here."

"You don't think that's just because we're in Sweden?" I ask. "Just last week Larry Kramer called them all murderers in his article in the *Village Voice*...."

"Yes, maybe you're right. Maybe when we go home we'll realize that it's still the same, but here, there's definitely a better feeling, a feeling of togetherness."

She goes on to say that she's in awe of the sexual openness of the Swedish society, and walks me over to the neighboring stand where dozens of sex education books are on display. "Do you know the story of the little rabbits?" Krim giggles and pulls one of the books off the rack. "There's this hilarious cartoon about the rabbits..." She shows me the cartoon. "They're in love, I think. I don't understand the story because it's in Swedish, but it's very funny." She points to one of the cartoons, one of a rabbit holding his genitals and looking sad. "Oy, oy, oy. Now what has happened to me?" Mathilde Krim roars with laughter.

The closing ceremony is identical to the opening one. A new collection of AIDS experts steps up to the podium to speak.

Outside, the weather in Stockholm is still perfect.

In a post-modern world that has largely lost traction with exacting language, the idea that there is *a* truth, that *something* is true, seems a tainted and suspect notion. All things are seen through the lens of an observer's ideological beliefs. What an observer thinks *should* be true. You could see this in the earliest attacks on Peter Duesberg, which came out primarily in left-leaning outlets, where Duesberg was pilloried, ridiculed, and finally completely ignored.

It seemed, in the early years, that Duesberg, by dissenting from the HIV theory, was making an attack on "lifestyle," since if AIDS wasn't caused by a novel and foreign retrovirus, it would have to be caused by other factors—perhaps one, as Duesberg often implied, having something to do with the history and behavior of a patient.

Despite the fact that the earliest attention to Duesberg and his conflicts with the HIV theory came from left-of-center outlets, the left cathedrals and many in the media insisted that the very idea of questioning HIV was inherently "right-wing" and pernicious. A scientist who argued that HIV did not cause AIDS became the incendiary equivalent to the religious right's primitive accusation that AIDS was God's punishment against homosexuals. All during these years, political correctness hung over America, leaving many Americans clear about what they could think, say, and publish. Duesberg's critique was never cast in the light of correct or incorrect, and few could be persuaded that Duesberg was not politically motivated. He was simply unable to tailor his inquiries or observations to suit the fashions of the times, and his scientific thinking was rarely described in the media with much accuracy.

It's doubtful that Duesberg even knew how his ideas would be received. Duesberg's questions, if one can put their scientific validity aside, did, more than anything, disrupt the calm that followed a government campaign which said that "HIV does not discriminate"—as pamphlets distributed by Surgeon General Koop to every single American household noted—a campaign that implied that the virus itself had undergone sensitivity training.

When pressed, by an increasingly hostile culture, to demonstrate what did cause AIDS, if not HIV, Duesberg made clear he was taking a shot, hazarding a guess, but was not sure. It was a hypothesis formed under intense pressure and out of necessity. Reviewing the literature closely, he settled on what was to him the most simple and obvious answer, if, to the world, the most infuriating and politically incorrect one: drugs. Around 1988, Duesberg set about documenting the final effect on the body's cellular system of a range of chemical assaults, from recreational to pharmaceutical. He picked up the CDC's own pre-HIV theory, which was that amyl nitrates—called "poppers" and used to facilitate anal sex in the bathhouses in the early 1980s—as well as scores of other drugs, could be causing the destruction of the immune system all by themselves. He began to collect data and write papers on this, which came to be known as the "Drug-AIDS hypothesis," but Duesberg himself admitted that he could neither prove or disprove his alternate theory without any funding to do so.

Originally, amyl nitrites were prescription drugs, used by the elderly for emergency relief of heart pain. It was not until the early '60s that gay men discovered new uses for the drugs. The FDA reinstated the prescription requirements for poppers in 1969 and in 1970, but manufacturers learned how to sidestep the FDA, marketing poppers as "room odorizers" and selling them directly to gay men, over the counter, from corner bodegas and newspaper shops. Poppers were the CDC's first embryonic AIDS causation theory, but they dismissed it quickly, when they became convinced that the "clustering" of AIDS could only be explained via sexual links, as many of the men who got sick were found to have had sex with one another. The CDC task force was stacked with Epidemic Intelligence Service officers, all of whom were searching out an infectious, rapidly spreading disease. To exonerate poppers, they cited a single study in mice, conducted in 1982-1983, claiming "no evidence of immunotoxicity" from poppers. However, this result was contradicted by other studies. One such study, conducted by Lee Soderberg of the University of Arkansas, found that mice exposed to poppers fumes for two weeks, forty-five minutes a day, had decreases in body and spleen weight, sharply reduced T-cells, and reduced white blood cell functions, among other effects. Later studies of poppers in mice showed that they also, with longer-term use, developed pneumonias and fungal infections. One study in HIV-negative gay men who inhaled poppers three times a day for a week concluded that "exposure to amyl nitrites can induce changes in immune function even after short exposure to moderate doses."

The details of Duesberg's theory about drugs and AIDS remain untested to this day, and it is the source of great frustration to Duesberg—to the chemist in him—that the effects of drugs on the human body are of no interest to the scientific community. He notes simply: "If you take Mercury, you get poisoned. If you take cyanide, you die. If you smoke cigarettes, you get emphysema. If you take nitrates, cocaine, heroin, and ·AZT, you're going to get sick. It's easy to test and understand. It's chemical toxicity. But there's no Nobel Prize in that, and that's why we don't want to look at it. No careers in it. It's truly 19th century science—and it's not attractive."

When Jon Cohen and *Science* magazine revisited Duesberg's questions about HIV and toxicity in the mid-'90s, Duesberg reiterated his interests in proving or disproving his toxicity hypothesis. His thinking, he claimed, could be confirmed or denied if other scientists would simply pay attention. He described modest experiments and studies to Cohen—including a study that would focus on hemophiliacs, a group that both Duesberg and his critics agreed would be an ideal test for his alternate explanation of AIDS. But Duesberg's experiments would not be tolerated, for by the time Duesberg started to examine and hypothesize about alternate causes of AIDS, he was already being accused of something new. Some scientists began saying that Duesberg's critique of the HIV hypothesis didn't amount to "falsifiable" theory, that is, it did not admit the possibility of being shown false and thus, according to rules laid out by Karl Popper in the 1930s, wasn't scientific. It was an accusation that stood in stark contrast to Duesberg—"the classical scientist"—who often described possible experiments to reporters and interested scientists.

As career damaging as it was to defend Duesberg, many colleagues from the highest ranks of classical virology did. These supporters included the renowned Berkeley virologist Harry Rubin, Nobel Laureates Walter Gilbert and Kary Mullis, and the legendary Yale mathematician Serge Lang. (Lang's tireless attempt to keep science from becoming politicized and distorted by the media continued until his death in 2005 and are catalogued in his book *Challenges*.) Rubin, Gilbert, Mullis, and Lang all fought for science itself when they argued that knowing whether Duesberg was right or wrong about his alternative ideas was not the point; the point was to defend Duesberg's right to challenge the orthodox view, propose an alternative, and be permitted to function as a scientist. But even these prestigious scientists were criticized.

In the March 1990 issue of the French journal *Research in Virology*, Dr. Luc Montagnier, whose lab at the Pasteur Institute in Paris first isolated HIV, reported that mycroplasma, a microbe with no cell wall, might be working in partnership with HIV to destroy human cells. It was one of the first discoveries that offered any hope of convincingly explaining how HIV was the trigger for AIDS.

In June of 1990, at the Sixth International Conference on AIDS in San Francisco, Montagnier planned to present his findings, which he believed suggested that mycroplasma microbes were a likely co-factor in the development of AIDS. The conference organizers offered fifteen minutes to Montagnier for his presentation. But fifteen minutes, Montagnier knew, wasn't enough. He arranged a longer opportunity to speak. As Elinor Burkett reported in the *Miami Herald*, Montagnier "planned to announce he had been wrong for almost seven years. He was about to explode a bomb in the midst of a multibillion-dollar international research and development establishment built on the bedrock truth he had helped create." Montagnier now believed HIV to be a "benign virus that only becomes dangerous in the presence of a second organism."

Montagnier stepped up to the microphone in San Francisco at a late-night conference session. Of the 12,000 conference attendees, 200 had shown up to see the discoverer of HIV, the scientist whose lab had set retroviral research on AIDS into motion. Montagnier, it was soon clear, was backing away from the accepted notion that HIV alone causes AIDS. His presentation revealed that the mycroplasma he had first announced in March were now responding to antibiotics in his lab. Although HIV kept replicating, without the mycroplasma, the cells that they infected stopped dying, in a test-tube in any case. Here was something new.

Although the implications for treatment promised to be enormous, for some reason, as he spoke, about half of those who had gathered to hear him simply left the auditorium.

One audience member who stuck around was Dr. Shyh-Ching Lo of the Armed Forces Institute of Pathology. He realized that Montagnier's mycoplasma was the same as the agent he had discovered in 1986. (And the same agent that he had presented at the International Conference on AIDS in 1988.) Montagnier's work, Lo quickly realized, independently confirmed his own results, and—with two serious studies on the topic completed, Montagnier's and his own—AIDS researchers would have to pay attention. Watching Montagnier's presentation in San Francisco, Lo was excited—his thinking about mycoplasma was about to go mainstream. Now a serious examination of mycoplasma would begin.

Lo's work on mycoplasma had already grown so detailed and promising that, in December of 1989, he had been invited to NIAID to discuss the topic. Most researchers there thought it would be easy to dismiss his work's relationship to AIDS outright. But, according the *Miami Herald*, scientists quizzed Lo for two days and soon realized why Lo was convinced of a connection: "'The documentation was absolutely solid,' said Joseph Tully, head of mycoplasma programs for NIAID. Participants formally recommended further study of the link between the mycoplasma and AIDS, and experiments with drugs that could kill the new microbe."

But in San Francisco, Jay Levy, a virologist at the University of California, San Francisco, and now considered one of the world's leading AIDS researchers, confronted Montagnier directly, arguing that he "had simply allowed his experiments to be contaminated—a mistake a graduate student might make." Levy insisted: "I've looked in twenty patients, and I can't find your mycoplasma." Montagnier calmly noted that the mycoplasma were "very hard to find." Levy responded angrily, saying, "We know how to look."

Levy, frustrated, turned his back on Montagnier and left the room. CDC spokesperson Peter Drotman later told the *Herald* that Montagnier's discovery was "just a hypothesis. We don't believe it. HIV is not a benign infection." When the *Herald* asked for comment on the bizarre and quick denouement, Peter Duesberg summarized: "There was Montagnier, the Jesus of HIV, and they threw him out of the temple." Montagnier, disgusted by the response of his American colleagues, left the conference early and flew back to Paris.

A day later, before any serious examination could be undertaken to examine Montagnier's results, the *New York Times* surveyed American AIDS researchers, who, in the main, responded as part of a chorus of denunciation. James Curran, then director of the AIDS program at the CDC, commented that he couldn't see the microbe "as a necessary co-factor, or the only co-facor." "Dr. Montagnier," he noted, "is really out on a limb."

Even through NIAID scientists recommended further study of Lo's mycoplasma, no such work was ever done. When the *Miami Herald* pressured Anthony Fauci, director of NIAID, to comment on the lack of research a year later, a spokesman responded that Fauci "will not talk about mycoplasma or any other AIDS co-factor." That Lo's work was now confirmed independently at the Pasteur

Institute made no difference. A day after Montagnier's presentation in San Francisco, Fauci still suspected contamination. He told the *New York Times* that, "There are enough gaps in the story that we can't get a clear understanding of it. It is still possible that this is due inadvertently to artifacts of the experiments."

The question of mycoplasma, however, eclipsed something much more substantial in Montagnier's presentation in San Francisco. His presentation chiefly raised repressed concerns about the cell-killing ability of HIV—concerns that, in many cases, closely echoed hesitations first expressed by Peter Duesberg. According to *Times* reporter Philip Hilts, "researchers have never understood why the AIDS virus is so lethal even with relatively little virus in the body. Dr. Montagnier suggested that another element is needed to change it into a killer.... These viruses 'normally live within the body, reproducing slowly over a long period without killing,' [Montagnier] said. 'It is not in the philosophy of retroviruses to kill the cells of the host.... We must explain why HIV is a killer virus. We tend to think of it as a slow virus. But in AIDS we some fast, highly pathogenic virus. The difference may be due to mycoplasma infection.'"

Montagnier was, of course, never entirely convinced of Gallo's claims about HIV. He once joking referred to the obscure source of the virus as "retroviral soup." As Dr. Etienne De Harven, a French virologist and pioneer of electron microscopy at Sloan Kettering, explained in an interview with me: "What the Pasteur team had in 1983—[which included] an excellent EM (electron microscopy) picture—demonstrates without any doubt that what they were looking at contained retroviruses budding on cell cultures. But their interpretation of that picture was that the lymphocytes had been infected by an exogenous virus, coming from the patient. They also said the culture was supplemented with normal human lymphocytes.... [the Pasteur team] had no grounds to use the word 'novel' for what they found." In other words, Montagnier and his French team had no reason to assume that "novel" invader virus might not turn out to be a previously unknown fragment of RNA.

In San Francisco, Montagnier was asking the establishment to consider the scientific problems tied to *assuming* that HIV alone causes AIDS. Robert Gallo had already, in a way, performed this feat in 1988 by claiming that the herpes virus HHV-6 was "definitely a co-factor in the development of AIDS." He may not have meant that HHV-6 was a necessary co-factor, but he implied that the virus might aid HIV. In reference to mycroplasma, Montagnier himself admitted that he had only a theory about how HIV might function—calling it an "extreme hypothesis that is reasonable." "If I cannot demonstrate it," Montagnier admitted, "I will go back to another hypothesis." Montagnier's search for a co-factor, however, was led by specific problems with the HIV hypothesis and could not be abandoned so easily. Speaking about HIV, the virus he had discovered, Montagnier insisted that a co-factor was necessary. To this day, Montagnier insists that HIV cannot lead to AIDS without other contributing causes.

The evidence supporting Montagnier's model of AIDS with more than one cause actually predates the discovery of HIV. One scientist in particular, Dr. Joseph Sonnabend, a researcher who had become a physician by the time AIDS began, worked during the early years of the epidemic to show that a handful of viruses can, by themselves, weaken the immune system to the point of collapse. Early on, his theory of AIDS and its accompanying evidence was in wide circulation; by May of 1983, *The Journal of the American Medical Association* published the first version of Sonnabend's hypothesis.

Sonnabend theorized that two specific stages lead to AIDS: the first stemming from accumulation of infectious assaults on the body. Repeated infection with CMV (cytomegola virus) and reactivation of EBV (Epstein-Barr virus), he noted, cause immune suppression, flu-like symptoms, and respiratory disease, all of which played an important role in the first stage. Multiple exposures to semen, Sonnabend also claimed, was dangerous, since foreign semen is immunosuppressive. Like blood, it carries tissue that is perceived as foreign when it comes into contact with another immune system and leads "to the appearance of antibodies reactive with an individual's T-lymphocytes." The second stage in Sonnaband's model was the complete breakdown of the immune system—or AIDS. Chief among Sonnabend's concerns was having an accurate model of AIDS sufficient for "prevention and intervention."

By 1983, Sonnabend had formed *AIDS Research*, the first medical journal to exclusively examine the epidemic. Sonnabend was in an unusual position to be able to study AIDS. He was a trained medical researcher, previously of London's National Institute for Medical Research, where he had worked with Alick Isaacs, the discoverer of interferon. He had also taught at the Mt. Sinai School of Medicine, Downstate Medical Center, and directed the Continuing Medical Education program at the Bureau of Venereal Disease Control for the New York City Department of Health. By the time AIDS hit, Sonnabend had opened a clinic in Greenwich Village to treat sexually transmitted diseases, and the large majority of his patients were gay. Unlike other AIDS scientists, in other words, he had a front row seat.

In *AIDS Research* in 1983, Sonnabend, because he had observed immuno-compromised patients, like transplant recipients, before AIDS began, proposed that there was "no specific etiologic agent of AIDS" and proposed once again that "the disease [AIDS] arises as a result of a cumulative process following a period of exposure to multiple environmental factors... The specific factors... are: (1) Immune responses to semen; (2) Repeated infections with cytomegalovirus (CMV); (3) Episodes of reactivation of Epstein Barr Virus (EBV); and (4) Infection with sexually transmitted pathogens, particularly those associated with immune complex formation such as Hepatitis B and Syphilis."

Sonnabend was also an early critic of Gallo's research. In 1982, when Gallo claimed in a paper that the HTLV-1 virus was related to AIDS, Sonnabend moved quickly to try to prevent the publication of Gallo's work. "It was absurd," Sonnabend remembered. "We could not find any trace of HTLV-1 in any tissue of AIDS patients, and yet Gallo was pushing this as the cause of AIDS. Nobody listened. Gallo had some kind of inexplicable power and influence, even then. Nobody wanted to go up against him." It was later clearly revealed that HTLV-1 was unrelated to AIDS. Sonnabend is also remembered, thanks to Randy Shilts' *And The Band Played On*, as the first scientist to be sure that Gallo had in fact appropriated HIV from the Pasteur Institute.

While Sonnabend didn't dispute the presence of HIV in AIDS patients, he had, over the many years he had treated AIDS, noticed a number of symptoms that he thought related. And yet, when Gallo made his famous announcement in 1984, related causes were no longer of interest to the medical community. "This whole HIV thing came like a monkey in the machinery," Sonnabend told me in 1988. "It's absolutely incomprehensible that this fraud was carried out in full public view.... It stopped everything and it's done everybody a great disservice."

Indeed, after Gallo's announcement in 1984, the crucial exploration of different co-factors that might be related to AIDS was entirely aborted. The synergy between an aggressive and highly motivated scientist, Gallo, a medical establishment desperate for a "quick fix" solution, and a surprisingly unscrutinizing press, all helped create the dogma that a single agent, HIV, causes AIDS. Investigations of other possible causes were abandoned, and government money and effort concentrated on HIV research exclusively. "If you get run over by a truck, you don't need co-factors," Gallo assured everyone.

In 1989, in light of wide assumptions about the etiologic role of HIV, Sonnabend revised his thesis about AIDS, noting that it would be wise to consider that "HIV is an effect, rather than a cause, of AIDS." Like Duesberg, Sonnabend questioned the cell-killing ability of HIV, but he also insisted that since a condition like AIDS was possible without HIV, researchers should be careful about attributing powers to HIV that could not be demonstrated by laboratory experiments. This was in an era when HIV's exact function was largely explained as "mysterious." Sonnabend insisted that since HIV had been circulating in the population for sometime, HIV could not be the only explanation for the widespread immune suppression known as AIDS. "Any hypothesis regarding the genesis of AIDS," Sonnabend insisted, "must explain why the syndrome has occurred at this time; in short, 'Why now?'"

Although Sonnabend's later work was done in partnership with government-funded researchers, his impressively argued model failed to gain support. He was never refuted; he was simply ignored.

He remained insistent, however, about his conclusions and multifactoral model, writing: "I have attempted to show why the contention that HIV causes AIDS should be returned to the realm of speculation. The costs of inappropriately accepting that the cause of AIDS has been firmly established to be HIV have been enormous, in time wasted and lives lost.... The cause or causes of AIDS remains unknown, and thus all hypotheses, including HIV, must be pursued."

After having conceded a prominent role for HIV in his multifactoral model, Gallo invited Sonnabend to the NIH to discuss AIDS related matters. Sonnabend, in an interview in *POZ* magazine, recalls the peculiar experience of being invited back into the establishment after having been thoroughly ignored: "During lunch, I was standing in line next to an NIH epidemiologist with whom I had interactions in the early days [of AIDS]. He turned to me and said, 'Oh, I guess it's OK to talk to you now.' It was a little joke. I mean, people shunned me. It was like little children, afraid to sit next to me or be seen talking to me." The joke, however, spoke volumes about AIDS research, for dissent from the HIV hypothesis simply wasn't tolerated.

Adding to the question of co-factors, John Maddox, the editor of *Nature*, sent shockwaves through the US and UK scientific communities in 1991 when he wrote an editorial essentially apologizing for not having given more credence to Duesberg's views about HIV. What prompted him, among other things, was a study that showed that mice, when injected with their own lymphocytes (immune system cells, of which T-cells are one class), may test positive for HIV antibodies despite never having been exposed to HIV. Maddox wrote, "Now there is some evidence to support [Duesberg's] long fight against the establishment (among which sadly he counts this journal)." He concluded his piece, which speculated that AIDS could be an autoimmune disorder, by saying that although he by no means feels that HIV is irrelevant to AIDS, the new research proves that AIDS is infinitely more complex than the original theory proposed. "Duesberg will be saying, 'I told you so,'" he wrote. The editorial was met with shock and outrage, and Maddox printed a partial retraction the next month, reassuring the scientific community that he was not saying he agreed with Duesberg about HIV, but that, as he said in a subsequent interview, there was more to AIDS than "baby-talk stories we've all been fed for years."

Indeed, if AIDS was more than "baby-talk stories," as Montagnier, Maddox, and Sonnabend all claimed, researchers had the chance to finally examine a more complicated understanding of AIDS. Such research might have also confirmed one of Duesberg's main hypotheses. In Duesberg's 1989 *PNAS* paper he noted that "Although HIV does not appear to cause AIDS, it may serve in the U.S. and Europe as a surrogate marker for the risk of AIDS." It wasn't, of course, that Duesberg denied any link between HIV and AIDS; rather, like the multifactoralist, he assumed that other factors were involved, and that HIV was indicative of those other, more active agents. For Duesberg's part, drug toxicity was the one that mattered. Others had different theories about other factors.

AIDS culture, however, allowed no dissent. And tragically, no serious study has ever been done to determine what factors, aside from HIV, AIDS patients have in common. It has been reported anecdotally, however, in testimonies from doctors with large AIDS practices and from AIDS support-group leaders, that those who come down with AIDS, like hemophiliacs and multiple-transfusion recipients, have a wide range of immuno-suppressive factors aside from HIV.

But because HIV is believed to cause death, we've always been left with a perpetual chicken-or-the-egg state of confusion. If HIV is present and death or disease occurs, HIV is held responsible. Rarely is the possibility considered that identical scenarios can take place without HIV—that all diseases associated with AIDS can occur on their own, particularly in already immune-compromised individuals. Various studies have reported on many cases of indisputable full-blown AIDS in which no trace of HIV could be found. How do the proponents of HIV explain cases like these? Their answer, especially in the early '90s, was simple, if unscientific: The virus is hiding. Indeed, every single discrepancy connecting the virus to AIDS is swept under the carpet with the explanation that the virus is simply mysterious, that it causes destruction silently, invisibly, inexplicably.

The year was 1987 and Duesberg had yet to announce his theory that drugs, pharmaceutical and recreational, cause AIDS. I was at an AIDS conference in Washington DC, having lunch at a diner, scribbling notes, my name tag hanging on my neck and identifying me as yet another earnest AIDS reporter. I was saved from a headlong fall into the politically correct version of the AIDS narrative then and there, I now realize, by a man seated in the next booth.

"You're an AIDS reporter?" he asked. He had a feline beauty about his face and looked right at me with green eyes, introducing himself as Michael Callen. "I can save you a lot of time," he said. "There is no parallel in your culture, in straight culture, for what goes on in the fast lane of gay life today. I have AIDS. To me, it is no mystery why I am sick but rather a miracle I am still standing. By the time I was twenty-five, I figure I had had sex with 3,000 people. I had had every STD you can imagine, several times, bacterial infections, parasitic infections... and unending rounds of antibiotics. This is not to speak of the drugs. There is no mystery here, about why we are getting sick. AIDS is a *multifactorial syndrome*, but straight people can't bring themselves to talk about what these factors are, and gay people don't want them to. We'll see if you're up to the task. I can tell you what you need to pursue."

"But let me warn you, this will not be a good career move. You will have your head handed to you."

Michael Callen, a thirty-three-year-old singer when I first met him, was a survivor. Six years after his diagnosis, he released his first solo album, *Purple Heart*, a collection of songs about being gay in the age of AIDS. By the time I met him, he had written and edited countless articles and books on AIDS, including the first explicit guide to safer sex. He co-founded the People with AIDS Coalition in New York and was a founding member of the National Association of People with AIDS. Callen had also helped launch the Community Research Initiative, an innovative group of bureaucracy-busters who got so fed up with federal indifference to AIDS that they rallied community doctors to start testing promising AIDS drugs themselves.

Callen told me his thinking about AIDS, influenced by his research and treatment, crystallized in two ways. First, he came to believe that AIDS patients could survive and thrive after prognosis. Early statistics confirmed that there were indeed long-term survivors; 15 percent of patients were living five years or longer in 1990, a statistic that would continue to rise as the epidemic went on. Callen advocated "hope," and he lectured around the country about how hope is indelibly connected to long-term survival. Second, he also realized, in partnership with his Greenwich Village physician, Dr. Joseph Sonnabend, that AIDS was caused by a long-term and multifactorial breakdown of the immune system.

Essentially, Michael Callen understood that he was living proof that surviving AIDS was possible. When he publicly announced that he had had AIDS for six years, many noted that such a survival rate wasn't possible, that Callen must have been misdiagnosed. "The notion is 'You have AIDS, you die.' If you don't die, that must mean you never had AIDS. That's the only explanation they're able to conceive of."

Micahel Callen's early emphasis on "hope" was tied to his observations about long-term survival, a possibility that was faintly apparent at the time, but which became more than obvious as the epidemic went on. In 1988, after profiling many long-term survivors, Callen framed his thinking in an interview with me: "Believing in the possibility of survival is one thing that ran through all the long-term survivors I interviewed. Despite all the propaganda, all the predictions from doctors, the deaths of all their other friends, each long-term survivor believed from the very beginning that they could survive. They found a way. They would either shut off the TV, or not read AIDS articles, which only talk about death, or not ask their doctors what their prognosis was. But without question, maintaining hope is the most important precondition for long-term survivors."

Early on it was said that a person would have no more than a year between infection with HIV and demise (it was even reported to be six months at one point). But the "latency period" grew fluidly and randomly, until it settled on between ten to fifteen years. Robert Gallo has even said that it "might be" up to thirty years in a healthy person. While many scientists state openly that HIV can take at least ten years to cause sickness, none has ever amended the death sentence that was originally handed down. Evidence also grew, and suppressed, of a large class of HIV-positive patients termed "long-term non-progressors," who test positive to HIV, have never take antiviral drugs, and show no signs of sickness. For example, in a question and answer forum online at an AIDS site at John's Hopkins Medical Center, a man named Gary wrote in saying he had been HIV positive and healthy for fourteen years. "Why hasn't anyone been curious to use me for some kind of research?" he asked the consulting doctor, Joel Gallant MD. The answer came back: "Gary, I don't want to burst your bubble, because you've obviously done very well, but what you're describing is not all that unusual. The AVERAGE time from infection to AIDS in an untreated person is ten years. That means that 50 percent of people will do better than that. In one study, it was estimated that 13 percent of gay men infected at a young age would remain symptom free for over twenty years, and that was before the days of protease inhibitors." It's an open secret now, but very few researchers are interested in survival. The overwhelming fear of HIV as a killer virus has made it difficult to have a rational debate on the issue, and the natural history of HIV positivity was rendered nearly impossible to observer once antiviral drugs became available.

In many ways, Callen's seemingly unscientific thinking about the epidemic reflected Luc Montagnier's less-than-orthodox position on the disease. In a 1997 interview with Djamel Tahi, Montagnier noted that "AIDS does not inevitably lead to death, especially if you suppress the co-factors that support the disease. It is very important to tell this to people who are infected. I think we should put the same weight now on the co-factors as we have on HIV. Psychological factors are critical in supporting immune function. If you suppress this psychological support by telling someone he's condemned to die, your words alone will have condemned him."

Callen also early on came out against use of AZT—saying that the risks of such a dangerous drug were outweighed by the evidence of long-term survival. Some critics of this cautious approach to AIDS treatment were particularly fierce. Martin Delaney, leader of the San Francisco AIDS group Project Inform, went so far as to state that Callen and Sonnabend, who shared Callen's thinking about AZT, were "complicit in the deaths of any AIDS patient who did not take AZT." Callen retorted at the time, "I am willing to accept the enormous responsibility for those patients if you will accept responsibility for those who *did* take AZT." Sonnabend invited Delaney, or anybody else, to go through his patient files and examine the last 100 deaths—when they were diagnosed, how long they survived, and what they finally died of—if a pro-AZT doctor would do the same. Nobody took him up on his challenge.

One of the most important contributions Callen and Sonnabend made to AIDS was also one of the most simple—at least it seems so now: safe-sex. But when they first proposed it in 1982, they were near crucified.

Callen, Sonnabend, and another of Sonnabend's patients, Richard Berkowitz, put their heads together and decided there was a politically safe thing to do and an ethically correct thing to do. They chose the later, and in 1982 Callen and Berkowitz wrote one of the most explosive and controversial articles ever published in the gay press. At a time when the gay sexual-liberation movement was still in full swing—when gay author Edmund White was declaring that "gay men should wear their sexually transmitted diseases like red badges of courage in a war against a sex-negative society"—an article was published in the *New York Native* that sent shockwaves through the community. It was titled "We Know

Who We Are: Two Gay Men Declare War On Promiscuity."

The point of the article was lost on most in the gay community, most of whom never forgave Callen or Berkowitz. It was a medical point, not a moral one, Callen remembered: "We were testifying about the urgent need to 'avoid the exchange of potentially infectious bodily fluids.'"

Members of GMHC (Gay Men's Health Crisis) and other critics felt that Callen and Berkowitz were "shouting guilt from the rooftops," and urging gay men to "follow along in self-flagellation."

"People actually thought I was blaming people for being sick," Callen noted. "I was naïve. I hadn't been political. I just thought, I'll write this and we'll have a much needed, long over-due debate. I thought most people would know I wasn't being moralistic, that I loved being a slut. But people were stunned. It was unfathomable. People walked up to me on the street and spat in my face."

The *New York Native* had initially agreed to run a follow-up article title "How to Have Sex in an Epidemic," but pulled out as a result of the controversy. "The second one was the important one," Callen told me. "The first one was rhetorical. It simply declared the problem. It said: There's an epidemic and we need to change how we have sex. The second part detailed *how* to change. How to *keep* having sex, only safely. But since the practical second part never followed, it came across as if in the middle of this crisis we were just smacking people, saying 'You boys have to stop.'"

Despite the controversy, which sparked explosive debates coast to coast, Callen persisted. In the end, he took his own tax-return money and published what became the first safe-sex manifesto: a forty-eight-page booklet titled *How to Have Sex in An Epidemic: One Approach*. The points put forth in the book have since become the nucleus of safe sex education programs throughout the world, including those of the once critical GMHC. Few remembered, or were ever told, how it started. "It was hard enough," Callen said, "to be sick and be freighted for my own life. To be attacked for trying to save the lives of others was deeply wounding. We were attacked by people whose advice was to play Donna Reed... to have fewer partners, whatever that meant, and to know your partners. But that advice was dangerously inadequate. I think the sense was that, just because a few of us died of a disease, it doesn't mean we have to stop the sexual revolution."

Callen and Berkowitz began their campaign against AIDS, of course, long before HIV was announced. Their belief in a multifactoral model led them to conceptualize an entire system of prevention that assumed many infectious agents, including CMV and the countless other diseases that AIDS patients were typically infected with. They kept open the possibility of a new virus, but for now targeted the many viruses and agents that they already new about and presumed to be involved in the many cases of AIDS they were watching around them. They wrote "if a new, as-yet-unidentified virus is responsible for AIDS, the measures proposed to prevent CMV transmission are likely to be effective in preventing the spread of any such virus.... What's over isn't sex—just sex without responsibility."

Theirs was a hard, if not impossible path. They were advocating a rigorous safe sex regimen reaching all areas of personal hygiene and avoiding STDs, and far more wide-ranging than the slogan others reduced their campaigns to: "use a rubber." "Gay men did a Queer Eye job on AIDS from the outset," complains Berkowitz, who is still alive today, more than twenty years after being delcared HIV-positive. "Gay men want things to be pretty, or to look pretty on the surface."

Callen managed to carry over his fight against AIDS into a

professional career as a singer and songwriter. He wrote the now famous AIDS anthem "Love Don't Need a Reason," which became the theme song for AIDS walkathons across the country, and "Living in Wartime," which was the opening song for Larry Kramer's Broadway play about AIDS, *The Normal Heart.*

As a scrupulous critic of both the medical establishment and the AIDS activist community's propaganda, Callen weathered countless attacks. Callen himself died in December 1993. He had survived full-blown AIDS for twelve years.

AIDS dissidents who pointed to a variety of questions about the HIV paradigm, including the possibility of surviving a positive HIV test or the importance of co-factors, were voracious readers, chroniclers, researchers, and collectors. I was often at gatherings and conferences with them in various corners of the world.

In 1992, dissidents gathered at a church in Amsterdam for a three-day conference called "AIDS: A Different View." The idea of the conference was that there was thinking about AIDS that was ignored by the media and among the speakers were Luc Montagnier and Peter Duesberg. Michael Callen and Joseph Sonnabend were also in attendance. The conference was organized by the Foundation for Alternative AIDS Research, a group of Dutch homeopaths who had decided that although only a minority held the view that that AIDS was not caused by HIV alone, the problems with the HIV hypothesis were substantial enough to merit serious attention. It was funded in part by the Dutch government and was the first public scientific forum on whether HIV was the only cause of AIDS. It was attended by some 200 delegates, including eminent scientists and many European journalists. There were, however, only two American journalists in attendance.

In his presentation, Montagnier reiterated his belief that one or several co-factors may "amplify" the disease process, but he emphasized that he did not agree with Duesberg that HIV is harmless. Montagnier did agree that Duesberg's main contention—that HIV does not kill cells—is correct, but he suggested that HIV proteins may trigger cell death at a later stage, which he believed could account for the depletion of immune system cells in people with AIDS. Montagnier also admitted that there were cases of AIDS without any trace of HIV. "We have to explain this," he said. "It's quite possible that some other agent sometimes introduces some kind of autoimmune reaction that destroys the immune system. HIV is not the only one."

The orthodox view in Amsterdam was represented by three Dutch AIDS researchers, Dr. Jaap Goudsmit, Dr. Roel Couthino, and Dr. Frank Miedema, who reiterated the case for HIV by pointing out that there is a near 100 percent correlation between HIV and AIDS. Couhino and Miedema both reported that they had done extensive studies on co-factors and their possible effects on AIDS progression and the studies had shown that co-factors were irrelevant.

But many were not persuaded by the presentation, in no small part because Goudsmit had recently been exposed for scientific fraud. In 1990, Goudsmit and a colleague, Henk Buck, had published a paper in which they claimed to have found a way to stop HIV from infecting cells. Goudsmit and Buck enjoyed a wave of fame and publicity until their claims underwent further examination. Separate panels found that the scientific methods used by Goudsmit were "misleading" and "poorly substantiated," and Buck's findings "bordered on fraud." In one case, according to *Science* magazine, they "carried out two identical experiments, but published only the one that supported their claims." Buck resigned and retracted his part of the work; no action was taken against Goudsmit.

Although the conference was at times ill-focused, it gave the skeptics a much needed opportunity to get together and compare notes. On the night before the conference, many dissidents sat down at a long wooden table in the basement of a hotel, together with the organizers of the conference. After a long and sometimes heated discussion, it was concluded that the one point on which all the HIV critics were united was that the final cause, or causes, of AIDS were not yet known. Not everyone agreed that HIV was *not* the cause of AIDS, but there was a strong consensus that it had not been conclusively proven.

Perhaps the most volatile issues at the conference was Duesberg's skepticism that AIDS was infectious. Duesberg's hypothesis led him to speculate that condoms were useless in preventing the spread of AIDS. It wasn't that Duesberg was against condom use so much as that he feared concentrating on safe-sex implied that AIDS had been proven infectious. Conference attendees fought bitterly over the safe sex question, dividing, finally, into two opposing factions, each of which fired off a release stating their position: One side said that Duesberg's statements on safe-sex were irresponsible and would "kill people"; the other, that Duesberg had a right to speak the truth as he saw it.

At the conference, Callen and Sonnabend, stood up and read a manifesto of sorts that they had penned, saying that Duesberg's statement that AIDS was not sexually transmitted was dangerous and had "threatened many lives." They were supported by others, many who questioned HIV, while believing that AIDS was, for sure, sexually transmitted, as had been demonstrated by the CDC.

The conference generated an unprecedented number of newspaper reports all over Europe and particularly in the UK. The London *Sunday Times* gave the HIV debate extensive coverage in the weeks leading up to the conference in a series of stories by Neville

Hodgkinson. Hodgkinson later told me that the articles drew significant protest, making it "very obvious that we've hit a nerve."

In the *Independent,* Dr. Dai Rees, the secretary of England's Medical Research Council, was quoted as saying that Duesberg's statements "represent a lethal cocktail of untruth and ignorance." An opinion piece by *Independent* science reporter Steve Connor equated believing Duesberg with "believing the world is flat."

Despite such dismissals by the press, the dissidents movement persisted. During the International Conference on AIDS in Geneva in 1998, the dissidents gathered in one of the city's underground bunkers. The lodgings for the dissidents at the conference had been arranged by two Swissair flight attendants, two gay men and came complete with full-body radiation suits hanging in the vestibule, and showers to wash off radiation. (Such bunkers, by law, existed beneath every single Swiss dwelling—in the unlikely event that Switzerland should be engaged in a nuclear war.) Dissidents including Huw Christie, Michael Baumgartner, Kevin Corbett, Claire Walton, and others felt the location fitting, as their counterparts in the orthodoxy were staying across town in four-star hotels.

But the early '90s would be the last time during which the causes of immunodeficiency besides HIV were fiercely debated in the mainstream. In January 1987, the FDA approved the drug AZT, and it was quickly taken up in the majority of media as a breakthrough in AIDS research. By the time the question of co-factors had arisen, drugs had taken center stage. By 1989, the AZT craze was in full swing, and the idea that antiviral drugs could bring an end to the AIDS plague was firmly established in the minds of AIDS doctors. A long line of antiviral remedies would follow. From this point on, the question of a co-factor, indeed any question about the cell-killing ability of HIV, simply fell away. A drug of some sort, it was widely assumed, would slay HIV and thus AIDS.

The demonstrated effectiveness of the drugs—according to an informal logic that soon went mainstream—meant that thinking about HIV must be correct.

In a certain sense, no researcher, not even Gallo, who proposed HHV-6 as a co-factor in 1988, or Montagnier, considering the role of mycoplasma in 1990, could stop this pharmaceutical charge. In 1997, Peter Duesberg ceased his AIDS research to return to his work on cancer. His theory that drugs contributed to AIDS was left untested, and his departure from AIDS research meant that the debate's central critic practically withdrew from mainstream debate about the question. In 1996, Robert Gallo departed the NIH amid questions of scientific misconduct relating to the isolation of HIV in his lab.

Doctors and researchers who continued to believe that AIDS was a multifactorial syndrome, or aided by co-factors were labeled "denialists," since any question about HIV's effect on the body was said to be "denying reality." Joseph Sonnabend's counterconventional approach to AIDS research lost him funding and the editorship of *AIDS Research*. The editorship went, in 1986, to Dani Bolognesi of Duke University, who had worked closely with Gallo on HIV. The journal was soon after renamed *AIDS Research and Human Retroviruses*, and the editorial board added staff from the NCI, NIH, and CDC, as well as Burroughs Wellcome, then the manufacturer of AZT.

More and more AIDS activists, beginning in 1987, turned almost exclusively to advocating for access to, and development of, antiviral drugs. The cause of AIDS, despite serious scientific questions on the part of many researchers, was fixed. HIV, the new ideology went, caused AIDS by itself. It was a deadly killer. No cofactor, indeed nothing beside HIV, was needed to cause AIDS. To this day, researchers have spent many billions of dollars on HIV research and practically nothing on alternative causes or co-factors.

It was at the International Conference on AIDS in Berlin in 1993 that I realized that the debate about drugs had overwhelmed AIDS research entirely. 1993 was the year of the so-called Concorde study on AZT—a vast and lengthy trial, the first not funded by the drug's maker—that showed that AZT was in fact shortening lives, as the so-called dissidents had long insisted. Because of this, there were a handful of dissidents who had made the pilgrimage to Berlin, each paying their own way—unlike the shouting, star players of such events, the representatives of ACT UP, who had been flown in first class and put up in fine hotels by various pharmaceutical companies.

It was also at the Berlin Conference that I joined television journalist Joan Shenton in the rescue of "Christian," a tall, skinny German man with long hair, bright green socks and white sneakers who'd been standing outside the conference center every day holding a handmade sign that read "Ab Zeum Teufel," with the letters AZT bolded: "To the devil—*AZT.*" He had been set upon by an angry mob of ACT UPers, beaten, his sign cracked in half, and his stack of anti-AZT flyers set on fire, as security guards watched.

The conference chair—a fat red faced German man—had incited this lynch mob mood, in his opening address, when he declared that there were some "deranged sociopaths," who did not believe that HIV was the cause of AIDS. He mentioned Peter

Duesberg by name and said he was insane and dangerous.

On the very first day of the conference, a Dutch man named Peter Laarhoven had deposited a stack of articles in the press room which quoted Luc Montagnier admitting he did not believe HIV alone caused AIDS. The articles were removed almost instantly, and Laarhoven himself was actually taken away by armed guards, one on each arm, and escorted off the premises. Then he was expelled from the country.

On a cold January day in 1987, inside one of the brightly-lit meeting rooms of the monstrous Food and Drug Administration (FDA) building, a panel of eleven top AIDS doctors pondered a very difficult decision. They had been asked by the FDA to consider giving lightning-quick approval to a highly toxic drug about which there was very little information. Clinically called Zidovudine, but nicknamed AZT after its components, the drug was said to have shown a dramatic effect on the survival of AIDS patients. The study that had brought the panel together had set the medical community abuzz. It was the first flicker of hope— people were dying much faster on the placebo than on the drug.

But there were tremendous concerns about the new drug. It had actually been developed a quarter of a century earlier as a cancer chemotherapy, but was shelved and forgotten because it was so toxic, expensive to produce, and totally ineffective against cancer. Powerful but unspecific, the drug was not selective in its cell destruction.

Drug companies around the world were sifting through hundreds of compounds in the race to find a cure, or at least a treatment, for AIDS. Burroughs Wellcome—then a subsidiary of Wellcome, a British drug company, and now part of the world's largest pharmaceutical company, GlaxoSmithKline—emerged as the winner. By chance, they sent the failed cancer drug, then known as Compound S, to the National Cancer Institute along with many others to see if it could slay the AIDS dragon, HIV. In the test tube at least, it did.

At the meeting, there was a lot of uncertainty and discomfort with AZT. The doctors who had been consulted knew that the study was flawed and that the long-range effects were completely unknown. But the public was almost literally baying at the door. Understandably, there was immense pressure on the FDA to approve AZT.

Everybody was worried about this one. To approve it, said Ellen Cooper, an FDA director, would represent a "significant and potentially dangerous departure from our normal toxicology requirements."

Just before approving the drug, one doctor on the panel, Calvin Kunin, summed up their dilemma. "On the one hand," he said, "to deny a drug which decreases mortality in a population such as this would be inappropriate. On the other hand, to use this drug widely, for areas where efficacy has not been demonstrated, with a potentially toxic agent, might be disastrous."

"We do not know what will happen a year from now," said panel chairman Dr. Itzhak Brook. "The data is just too premature, and the statistics are not really well done. The drug could actually be detrimental." A little later, he said he was also "struck by the facts that AZT does not stop deaths. Even those who were switched to AZT still kept dying."

"I agree with you," answered another panel member. "There are so many unknowns. Once a drug is approved, there is no telling how it could be abused. There's no going back."

Burroughs Wellcome reassured the panel that they would provide detailed two-year follow-up data, and that they would not let the drug get out of its intended parameters: as a stopgap measure for very sick patients. Dr. Brook was not won over by the promise. "If we approve it today, there will not be much data. There will be a promise of data," he predicted, "but then the production of data will be hampered."

"There was not enough data, not enough follow-up," Brook told me in 1989. "Many of the questions we asked the company were answered by, 'We have not analyzed the data yet,' or 'We do not know.' I felt that there was some promising data, but I was very worried about the price being paid for it. The side effects were so very severe. It was chemotherapy. Patients were going to need blood transfusions. That's very serious."

"The committee was tending to agree with me that we should wait a little bit, be more cautious," Brook remembered. "But once the FDA realized we were intending to reject it, they applied political pressure. At about 4 p.m., the head of the FDA's Center for Drugs and Biologics asked permission to speak, which is extremely unusual. Usually they leave us alone. But he said to us, 'Look, if you approve the drug, we can assure you that we will work together with Burroughs Wellcome and make sure the drug is given to the right people.' It was like saying 'please do it.'"

Brad Stone, FDA press officer, was at that meeting. He has said he doesn't recall that particular speech, but that there is nothing "unusual" about FDA officials making such speeches at advisory meetings. "The people in that meeting approved the drug because the data the company had produced proved it was prolonging life. Sure it was toxic, but they concluded that the benefits clearly outweighed the risks."

When the 1987 meeting ended, AZT was approved, although several members of the panel feared it could be a time bomb. Dr. Itzhak Brook's vote was the only one cast against approval.

The majority of those in the AIDS-afflicted and medical communities held the drug up as the first breakthrough in AIDS. For better or worse, AZT had been approved faster than any drug in FDA history, and activists considered it a victory. The price paid for victory, however, was that almost all government drug trials focused on AZT—while over 100 other "promising drugs" were left uninvestigated.

Burroughs Wellcome stock went through the roof when the announcement was made. At a price of $8,000 per patient per year (not including blood work and transfusions), AZT was, at the time, the most expensive drug ever marketed. Burroughs Wellcome sold $159 million worth of AZT in 1988, with sales reaching $200 million by 1989. Wellcome was reportedly making 80 percent gross profit margin on the drug's sale. In the late '80s, stock market analysts widely and publicly speculated about Burroughs Wellcome profitability, assuming that, because of expanded prescription, the drug would become the largest share of Wellcome's profits by the mid-'90s.

AZT was the only antiretroviral drug that received FDA approval for treatment of AIDS from 1987 until 1991, and the decision to approve it was based on a single study that has long been declared invalid. The study was intended to be a "double-blind placebo-controlled study," the only kind of study that can effectively prove whether or not a drug works. In such a study, neither patient nor doctor is supposed to know if the patient is getting the drug or a placebo. In the case of AZT, the study became unblinded on all sides, after just a few weeks.

Many factors contributed to the unblinding. It became obvious to doctors who were getting what, because AZT caused such severe side effects which AIDS per se did not. Furthermore, a routine blood count, which clearly showed who was on the drug and who was not, wasn't whited out in the reports. Both of these weaknesses were accepted and confirmed at the time by both the FDA and Burroughs Wellcome, who conducted the study. Indeed, many of the patients who were in the trial admitted that they had analyzed their capsules to find out whether they were getting the drug. If they weren't, some bought the drug on the underground market. Also, pills were supposed to be indistinguishable by taste, but they were not. Although this was corrected early on, the damage was already done. There were early press reports that patients were pooling pills out of solidarity with each other. The study was so severely flawed that its conclusions should have been considered, by the most basic scientific standards, unproven.

The most serious problem with the original study, however, was that it was never completed. Seventeen weeks into the study, when more patients had died in the placebo group, than in the group on AZT, the study was stopped short, and all subjects were put on AZT.

Dr. Brook warned at the time that AZT, being the only drug available for doctors to prescribe to AIDS patients, would probably have a runaway effect. Approving it prematurely, he said, would be like "letting the genie out of the bottle." Brook pointed out that since the drug is a form of chemotherapy, it should only be prescribed by doctors who have experience with chemotherapeutic drugs. Because of the most severe toxic effects of AZT— cell depletion of the bone marrow—patients would need frequent blood transfusions. As it happened, AZT was rampantly prescribed as soon as it was released, way beyond its purported parameters and the worst-case scenario had come true: Doctors interviewed by the *New York Times* late in 1987 revealed that they were already giving AZT to healthy people who had tested positive for antibodies to HIV.

The FDA's function is to weigh a drug's efficacy against its potential hazards. The equation is simple and obvious: A drug must unquestionably repair more than it damages, otherwise the drug itself may cause more harm than the disease it is supposed to fight.

AZT was singled out among hundreds of compounds when Dr. Sam Broder, then head of the National Cancer Institute, found that it "inhibited HIV viral replication in vitro." AZT was thought to work by interrupting DNA synthesis, thus stopping further replication of the virus. While it was always known that the drug was exceedingly toxic, the first study concluded that "the risk/benefits ratio was in favor of the patient." In the study that won FDA approval for AZT, the one fact that swayed the panel of judges was that the AZT group outlived the placebo group by what appeared to be a landslide. The ace card of the study, the one that cancelled out the issue of the drug's enormous toxicity, was that nineteen persons had died in the placebo group and only one in the AZT group. The AZT recipients were also showing a lower incidence of opportunistic infections.

While the data staggered the panel that approved the drug, other scientists insisted that it meant nothing—because it was so shabbily gathered, and because of the unblinding. Shortly after the study was stopped, the death rate accelerated in the AZT group. "There was no great difference after a while," recalled Dr. Brook, "between the treated and the untreated group."

The scientific facts about AZT and AIDS were indeed astonishing. Most ironically, the drug had been found to accelerate the very process it was said to prevent: the loss of T-4 cells. In actual fact, AZT kills T-4 cells, white blood cells vital to the immune system. Critics of the drug pointed out that it was a "chain-terminating nucleotide," which dangerously interrupted the process of DNA replication. In the late '80s, when specific questions about the alleged mechanisms of AZT were asked, the answers came long, contradictory, and riddled with unknowns. Every scientific point raised about the drug was eventually answered with the blanket response, "The drug is not perfect, but it's all we have right now." About the depletion of T-4 cells and other white cells, Burroughs Wellcome scientists Sandra Lehrman said, "We don't know why T-4 cells go up at first, and then go down. That is one of the drug mechanisms that we are trying to understand."

The toxic effects of AZT, particularly bone marrow suppression and anemia, were so severe that up to 50 percent of all AIDS patients could not tolerate it and had to be taken off it. In the approval letter that Burroughs Wellcome sent to the FDA, all of fifty additional side effects of AZT, aside from the most common ones, were listed. These included: loss of mental acuity, muscle spasms, rectal bleeding, and tremors.

Severe anemia, one of AZT's common side effects, means the deficiency of red blood cells, but without red cells, you cannot pick up oxygen. Fred, a person with AIDS, was put on AZT and suffered such severe anemia from the drug that he had to be taken off it. In an interview in Michael Callen's AIDS handbook *Surviving and Thriving With AIDS*, Fred described what his severe anemia felt like in 1987: "I live in a studio and my bathroom is a mere five-step walk from my bed. I would just lie there for two hours; I couldn't get up to take those five steps. When I was taken to the hospital, I had to have someone come over to dress me. It's that kind of severe fatigue.... The quality of my life was pitiful.... I've never felt so bad.... I stopped the AZT and the mental confusion, the headaches, the pains in the neck, the nausea, all disappeared within a twenty-four-hour period."

"I feel very good at this point," Fred went on. "I feel like the quality of my life was a disaster two weeks ago. And it really was causing a great amount of fear in me, to the point where I was taking sleeping pills to calm down. I was so worried. I would totally lose track of what I was saying in the middle of a sentence. I would lose my directions on the street."

Jerome Horowitz, the man who invented AZT, commented in 1989 that "Yes, AZT is a form of chemotherapy.... It is cytotoxic, and as such, it causes bone marrow toxicity and anemia. There are problems with the drug. It's not perfect. But I don't think anybody would agree that AZT is of no use. People can holler from now until doomsday that it is toxic, but you have to go with the results."

But the results, finally and ironically, were what damned AZT. Several studies on the clinical effects of AZT—including the one that Burroughs Wellcome's approval was based on—have drawn the same conclusion: that AZT was effective for a few months, but after that its effect drops off sharply. Even the original AZT study showed that T-4 cells went up for a while and then plummeted. HIV levels went down, and then came back up. This fact was well known when the FDA advisory panel voted for approval. As panel member Dr. Stanley Lemon said in the meeting, "I am left with the nagging thought after seeing several of these slides, that after sixteen to twenty-four weeks—twelve to sixteen weeks, I guess—the effect seems to be declining."

A follow-up meeting, two years after the original Burroughs Wellcome study, was scheduled to discuss the long-range effects of AZT, and the survival statistics. Burroughs Wellcome made the claim that AZT lowered the level of HIV in the blood—measured by an antigen called p24. At the first FDA meeting, Burroughs Wellcome emphasized how the drug had "lowered" the p24 levels; at this follow-up meeting, they didn't mention it. (As one doctor present at that meeting in May 1988 recalled, "They hadn't followed up the study. Anything that looked beneficial was gone within half a year. All they had were some survival statistics averaging forty-four weeks. The p24 didn't pan out, and there was no persistent improvement in the T-4 cells."

"What counts is the bottom line," one of the scientists representing Burroughs Wellcome summed up, "the survival, the neurologic function, the absence of progression and the quality of life, all of which are better. Whether you call it better because of some antiviral effect, or some other antibacterial effect, they are still better."

"There have always been drugs that we use without knowing exactly how they work," commented Nobel Prize winner Walter Gilbert. "The really important thing to look at is the clinical effect. Is the drug helping or isn't it?"

The last surviving patient from the original AZT trial, according to Burroughs Wellcome, died in 1989. When he died, he had been on AZT for three and one-half years. He was the longest surviving AZT recipient. The longest surviving AIDS patient overall, not on AZT, had, at the time, lived for eight and one-half years.

In the early days, AZT was said to extend lives. In actual fact, there was simply no solid evidence that it did.

But the truth about AZT did not penetrate the media quickly. Most facts about AZT had a tortuous history: A number of studies confirming what could have already been understood in 1987 only slowly came to light. In December 1988, a study was published in the *The Lancet* that Burroughs Wellcome and the NIH did not include in their press kits. It was more expansive than the original AZT study and followed patients longer. It was not conducted in the United States, but in France, at the Claude Bernard Hospital in Paris, and concluded the same thing about AZT that Burroughs Wellcome's study did, except Burroughs Wellcome called their results "overwhelmingly positive," while the French doctors called theirs "disappointing." The French study found, once again, that AZT was too toxic for most to tolerate, had no lasting effect on HIV blood levels, and left the patients with fewer T-4 cells than they started with. Although they noticed a clinical improvement at first, they concluded that "by six months, these values had returned to their pretreatment levels and several opportunistic infections, malignancies, and deaths occurred."

"Thus the benefits of AZT are limited to a few months for ARC [AIDS-related complex] and AIDS patients," the French team concluded. After a few months, the study found, AZT was completely ineffective.

On August 17, 1989, newspapers across America bannerheadlined that AZT had been "proven to be effective in HIV antibody-positive, asymptomatic and early ARC patients," even though one of the FDA panel's main concerns was that the drug should only be used as a last-case scenario for critically-ill AIDS patients, due to the drug's extreme toxicity. NIAID head Dr. Anthony Fauci was now pushing to expand prescription.

The FDA's concerns had been thrown to the wind. Already the drug had spread to sixty countries and an estimated 20,000 people. Not only had no new evidence allayed the initial concerns of the panel, but the follow-up data, as Dr. Brook predicted, had fallen by the wayside. The beneficial effects of the drug had been proven to be temporary. The toxicity, however, stayed the same.

The government announced that an estimated 1.4 million healthy, HIV antibody-positive Americans could "benefit" from taking AZT, even if they showed no symptoms of disease. New studies, according to press reports, had "proven" that AZT was effective in stopping the progression of AIDS in asymptomatic cases. Dr. Fauci proudly announced that a trial that had been going on for "two years" had "clearly shown" that early intervention would keep AIDS at bay. Anyone who had antibodies to HIV and less than 500 T-4 cells should start taking AZT at once, he said. In 1988, this was approximately 650,000 people in the U.S. The rest of the 1.4 million Americans then assumed to be HIV-positive may also need to take AZT so they don't get sick, Fauci contended.

The leading newspapers didn't seem to think it unusual that there was no existing copy of the study, but rather only a breezy two-page press release from the NIH. According to the study, 3,200 asymptomatic patients were divided into two groups, one AZT and one placebo, and followed for two years. The two groups were distinguished by T-4 cell counts; one group had less than 500, the other more than 500. These two were then divided into three groups each: high-dose AZT, low-dose AZT, and placebo. In the group with more than 500 T-4 cells, AZT had no effect. In the other group, it was concluded that low-dose AZT was the most effective, followed by high-dose. All in all, thirty-six out of 900 developed AIDS in the two AZT groups combined, and thirty-eight out of 450 in the placebo group. "HIV-positive patients are twice as likely to get AIDS if they don't take AZT," the press release declared.

The study boasted that AZT was much more effective and less toxic at one-third the dosage than had been used for three years. That was the good news. The bad news was that thousands had already been walloped with 1,500 milligrams of AZT and had died of toxic poisoning.

On April 5, 1990, a full nine months after the NIH announced to the public that anyone with antibodies to HIV and less than 500 T-4 cells should start taking AZT, the study behind this policy was made public. The results of the study were published in the *New England Journal of Medicine*, but the details came too late. By the time the actual study was made public, labs on the West Coast and in Europe were reaching quite different conclusions. Investigators at the Veterans Administration (VA) and in Europe had also administered AZT in asymptomatic patients over a period of two years and in the March 23, 1990, *JAMA* (*Journal of the American Medical Association*) it was reported that they had "not seen benefit in such patients. . . ."

John D. Hamilton, MD, co-chair of the VA study, said analysis at two years demonstrated "no statistical difference in progression to AIDS," and that deaths in both placebo and AZT groups were "virtually identical." The article continued that "thoughtful, intelligent and ethical physicians" may want to let stable patients with T-cell counts closer to 500, a standardized threshold for failing immunity, "choose not to take the drug."

But then came August 1993 and what is remembered as "official" confirmation of what had been known for years: the Anglo-French "Concorde" study. Concorde went on for three years, examining 1,749 HIV-positive but healthy people at thirty-eight health centers in the U.K., Ireland, and France. Because the research lasted the longest of all AZT studies, and its pedigree was unassailable (it was conducted by the highly reputable British Medical Research Council and its French equivalent), Concorde could not be dismissed. The team concluded that AZT neither prolongs life nor staves off symptoms of AIDS in people who are HIV-antibody positive but healthy.

The preliminary results of the study were announced at Ninth International AIDS Conference in Berlin. Rumors circulated around the conference that the Concorde team had been under tremendous pressure from AZT's manufacturer to soften its results. After one of the sessions in which the results were discussed, I walked up to Dr. Ian Weller, a chief investigator of Concorde, and I asked whether there had indeed been pressure from Wellcome. He nodded.

A woman standing next to him, also on the Concorde team, nodded emphatically and finally burst out: "Yes, there has been pressure, and it has been placed at the very highest level."

She looked at me with a very pained expression on her face and said, rather quietly: "The most frustrating thing is that I can't tell you about it."

Weller cleared his throat. "We've carried out this study against incredible adversity, but we are not going to cave in to any pressure," he said. "We'll win the battle in the end. We show the science, that's all that matters."

I asked him how he felt about the fact that doctors in the U.S. still prescribed AZT to asymptomatics. "I think Concorde is going to take time to sink in," he said. "How you take on board the results very much depends on what you believe in before you saw them." As an afterthought he added, "I think it's very hard, if you've been giving AZT to large numbers of patients, to swallow this result."

More ominous than 1993's Concorde report was the study by Dr. Jens Lundgren and colleagues published in the April 1994 issue of the *JAMA* suggesting that the use of AZT actually shortens life. The study, conducted at fifty-one centers in seventeen European countries, compares patients treated and not treated with AZT. Like the Concorde study, the Lundgren research was revealing because it did what none of the original AZT studies did: It looked at the long-term results. Virtually every U.S. AZT study was terminated prematurely as soon as "survival benefit" was observed. The Lundgren study persevered for five years. A total of 4,484 patients were observed who had been diagnosed with AIDS during the '80s and who had not taken AZT before the trial. Among the patients who stayed off the drug, the death rate was approximately constant for the first five years after diagnosis.

For those who did take AZT, there was an upswing followed by a nosedive. The death rate in the third and forth years was "substantially greater" than for those who never took the drug.

The study received no major media play in the U.S., nor did the activist community vent any rage. TAG's (Treatment Action Group) Spencer Cox explained: "We're not interested in culpability right now. We'll get to that later, when there's time. Right now we have to figure out what works."

But the 1994 study concluded what skeptics had argued for years: That the slight benefits of taking the drugs are often canceled out by the many, severe side effects.

It's 1998. Kris Chmiel is a housewife and mother of two young children, living in Denver. In 1996, when she was pregnant with her second child, a movement had just gotten under way to test all pregnant women in the state of Colorado for HIV. She was perfectly healthy and in her first month of pregnancy. She wasn't worried—she had been monogamous with her husband for the past nine years. When the test came back "positive," she literally did not believe it.

Her doctors strongly urged her to immediately start taking AZT in an effort to prevent transmission to her child. "They finally wore me down," she says, "even though it was totally against my intuition."

In her fifth month of pregnancy, Chmiel began taking 500 milligrams of AZT, which was routinely prescribed to pregnant HIV-positive women following a 1994 study—ACTG 076—which claimed efficacy in reducing the transmission from mother to child. While AZT was shown to be ineffective for long-term treatment of AIDS patients, the drug was re-launched as an "effective" way to prevent passing HIV from mother to child.

Chmiel's daughter was two-years-old in 1998 and had twice tested negative for HIV infection. By the standards of the AIDS establishment, she was not only a success story, but the very epitome of medicinal victory. She was precisely the kind of baby who would serve as a poster child for mandatory testing, as well as mandatory treatment—a "saved" baby.

But to Chmiel, there were strong undertones of regret, anger, and even despair when she looked back on her choice to take AZT. Follow-up HIV tests after her child was born gave results different from the first one, throwing into question whether she ever did have HIV. One test was indeterminate, and another was negative. She soon started doing her own research, and found a paper citing all the underlying conditions—as many as sixty-four—that can cause a false positive HIV-antibody test. One of them is pregnancy.

She also became more and more aware of the potential toxic effects of AZT. There are five categories that the FDA uses for pregnancy drug classification, listed from the safest to most dangerous—A, B, C, D, and X. AZT is listed in Category C and is described as a drug in which "safety in human pregnancies has not been determined, animal studies are either positive for fetal risk or have not been conducted, and the drug should not be used unless the potential benefit outweighs the potential risk to the fetus."

For Chmiel, who stayed on AZT for a year after her child was born, the breaking point with AZT came when the drug's toxicity became so overwhelming that she crawled to the bathroom and kept vomiting for hours. "I just couldn't take it anymore," she said, adding that when she stopped taking the drug, her health returned.

Many studies have noted that an increasing number of children born HIV-positive are growing into adolescence without any sign of sickness. A study that came out of the

1996 International AIDS Conference in Vancouver reported that 37 percent of all HIV- positive babies would never progress into full-blown AIDS. In his 1993 book *Rethinking AIDS*, Robert Root-Bernstein states, "Less than a third of HIV-sero-positive infants go on to develop AIDS."

It may be nearly impossible to ferret out what precisely we mean when we talk about children "progressing," because the waters are clouded from the start. Progressing from what to what? As Root- Bernstein points out in his book, 80 percent of HIV-positive infants in the U.S. in 1993 were born to drug-addicted mothers—whose immune systems are severely compromised with or without HIV—and those babies all will inherit their mother's immune system. If the mother is sick, the baby will be sick. Unfortunately, few research efforts have been aimed at truly resolving the fundamental question of how HIV, as distinct from all other factors, affects children, because mainstream HIV dogma holds that there is no question.

"Do you think that AZT had any adverse effect on your child?" I ask Chmiel.

"Yes, I do," she says firmly. "She has a very enlarged cranium. That's typical of most of the AZT babies I have observed."

"They're killing babies," she says emphatically. She cites a young woman who came to her for counseling at the dissident AIDS activist group HEAL in Denver, who had watched her child test positive for HIV shortly after being vaccinated (vaccinations can cause the HIV test to produce a false positive). The baby was put on AZT, despite the fact that the mother was HIV-negative. Three months later, the baby was dead. Another mother who contacted Chmiel had a baby with hemophilia, who had received Factor 8 clotting plasma (yet another possible source of false positives). After testing positive, the baby was put on several medications and died after only five months. "That child's mother is still devastated," Chmiel says. "She believes it was the drugs that killed her son."

Even when children taking AZT survive, Chmiel firmly believes, the consequences of the drug use can be dire. "I went to this conference that they held on HIV and pregnancy at Children's Hospital here in Denver," she says, "and a lot of the mothers there had taken AZT during pregnancy, and they had their kids with them. I looked from one to the other, and every single one of those kids had enlarged craniums. Their heads looked exactly like my kid's head. They're all AZT babies."

Few, if any, studies in the history of AIDS research have caused such a momentous shift in policy, medical practice, and zeitgeist as the one called ACTG 076. To believers, it was perhaps the single greatest breakthrough in the history of AIDS research, but to its detractors, it was the most alarming and radical turn prenatal care has ever taken.

If you called up virtually anybody who worked within obstetrics, HIV/AIDS, and pediatrics during the late '90s, they would have told you the same thing: that the protocol now known simply as 076—the study that first caused the FDA to approve the use of AZT in pregnant women—has been perhaps the most unequivocally encouraging news in all of HIV/AIDS research. Fourteen hundred babies per year in the United States alone, most claimed, were "saved" by AZT use, which by unknown mechanisms is said to reduce maternal transmission of HIV. Most would have also have told you that there had been no documented complications from AZT, and that even if there were, they paled in comparison to the dreadful effects of HIV itself.

In ACTG 076, the transmission of HIV during labor was reduced from 25.5 percent in the placebo group to 8.3 percent in the group that was given AZT throughout the second and third trimesters and intravenously during labor. The babies in that group were then given AZT for six weeks after birth. Maternal transmission rates vary greatly—in industrialized countries, 25 percent is certainly the high end. In several European studies, the rate is as low as between about 7 percent and 14 percent—levels that are said to correlate with improved prenatal care. In one quite surprising study from Malawi, it was found that transmission was closely correlated with levels of vitamin A in the mother. Those with the lowest levels transmitted HIV to their babies at a rate of 32.4 percent, while those with the highest levels had a transmission rate of only 7.2 percent—a figure lower than the lowest figures attributed to AZT. And yet, the discourse around this subject is framed inextricably around the notion that toxic medications constitute the only legitimate and, for the mother, "responsible" route to reduced transmission.

Such pharmaceutical intervention during pregnancy is obviously a major shift in policy. Following recent disasters—remember thalidomide?—the FDA imposed far stricter regulations on what women could be exposed to while pregnant—essentially nothing. Thalidomide, of course, was prescribed as a sedative in both Great Britain and Europe in the 1950s. Years later, it was found to have caused at least 10,000 severe birth defects. Not too long afterward, DES, a synthetic hormone that was prescribed to women in the 1940s and 1950s to prevent miscarriages, was found to be causing vaginal cancer in the daughters of the women who had taken it during pregnancy.

These two catastrophes produced a powerful impact on both the public and the medical community, resulting in a total ban on exposing women to chemicals during pregnancy. In 1990, however, ACTG 076 broke that policy, opening the medical floodgates for the chemically promiscuous scenario that we have today, in which pregnant women are given not just AZT, but multiple combinations of other drugs—including protease inhibitors—aimed at reducing "viral load" of HIV.

This extreme break in policy can only be explained by the climate of AIDS and HIV, which dictates that no measure is too extreme, or too risky, if it results in the perceived diminishment of HIV transmission. UNICEF and the World Health Organization (WHO) launched drives to get AZT distributed to all pregnant HIV-positive women in developing countries. But since they lacked the facilities for proper HIV testing, the only possible scenario was for AZT to be handed out indiscriminately. When the plan was first unveiled years ago, Laurie Garrett, a reporter for New York *Newsday*, speculated that, not knowing which women are truly infected and which are not, "They would have no other choice but to treat every woman in labor with the chemical."

This speaks volumes about the decline of critical thinking in the era of AIDS—it is now considered reactionary, even outright "irresponsible," to question the wisdom of exposing pregnant women to such a wide array of mutagenic, carcinogenic, teratogenic agents.

It is common today for AZT to be referred to as "safe" for pregnant women. But the FDA never considered it so before and banned pregnant HIV-positive women from taking it, prior to 076. AZT was classified as a mutagenic agent, which thalidomide also is, and the controversy in the early days of AIDS—the activist outcry—was that women were being excluded from all clinical AIDS drug trials. Indeed they were—the FDA was rightly concerned about the possible effects of these potent drugs on future babies.

ACTG 076, which was funded in part by AZT's maker, then Glaxo-Wellcome, was designed to determine whether treating pregnant, HIV-positive women with AZT during pregnancy would reduce the rate of HIV transmission from mother to child. That was the first objective. The second, strangely enough, was to see whether AZT is safe—for mother or for child. An 076-trial memo stated that, "although safety [is] unknown it can be argued that any possibility of stopping transmission to the fetus outweighs perceived risks to the woman."

"You have to put all this into a framework," noted Kathleen Nokes, an RN and a project director of Nursing Persons With HIV/AIDS. "Many people are angry that these women are getting pregnant. So it's like, 'Well, if the mother is going to have this baby, we will have to intervene to protect it.' That is the mind-set. And the intervention is AZT."

This despite the fact that criticisms have been made of the design and the conclusions of 076. The study's authors themselves, when they reported their findings in the *New England Journal of Medicine* in 1994 admitted that the efficacy of AZT in reducing maternal transmission of HIV is "impossible to quantify [absolutely] because of the very small numbers of infected babies [studied]." They also noted that the rate of the HIV transmission in the placebo group was inexplicably high.

And could the results be repeated? It is impossible to say, since the "overwhelming" results of 076 rendered it "unethical" to ever again use a placebo control group. In fact, when it later came to light that studies using placebo controls were underway in Thailand and Africa, there was an uproar in the medical community that was so loud that several editors from the *NEJM* quit their jobs over the perceived immorality of the trials. A preliminary report from the trial in Thailand, however, showed no difference between the group treated with AZT and the placebo group in terms of transmission rates.

Like so many of the studies involving AZT, ACTG 076 was terminated as soon as a benefit was seen on the AZT side. At the study's first interim analysis, thirteen babies (8.3 percent) in the AZT group were reported to be HIV-positive, versus forty (25.5 percent) in the placebo group. A total of 477 women were recruited for the study.

The popular media trumpeted the news that the discredited AIDS drug AZT had made an astonishing comeback in a patient group that had previously been exiled from clinical trials. It was as if the medical community was honoring women by including them. The Clinton administration touted the study's surprising results as proof of an unprecedented breakthrough in AIDS. A kind of wild D-Day euphoria spread through the OB-GYN community, which now finally had something hopeful to tell pregnant HIV-positive mothers. This "science by press release" took hold before any independent review board had verified the data, and nine months before the study itself was published.

Eventually it came to light that the doctor who had leaked the ACTG 076 story to the *New York Times* was a paid consultant to the drug's maker, then Glaxo-Wellcome. Still, the influential U.S. Pediatric AIDS Foundation, now the Elizabeth Glaser Pediatric AIDS Foundation, and many other pediatric institutions, immediately announced that all HIV-infected women should be offered AZT, and that this "lifesaving treatment cannot be ethically denied because of ineffective HIV screening."

AZT has been approved for use not only in pregnant HIV-positive women, but also in newborns, for whom there previously had been no "standard of care."

"They have progressed from basic research to 'standard of care' so fast," said Nokes. "And once it is standard care, that's that.

If we prescribe AZT to your baby, and you don't give it to her, we take you to court for child abuse."

Many women have had precisely this nightmarish experience.

Jenny Guembes, an HIV-positive mother of a healthy seven-year-old boy, counseled HIV-positive women for the AIDS Healthcare Foundation in Los Angeles. "When these pregnant women come here, I tell them, 'Look, if you have a low viral load, there's a good chance you won't transmit.' I tell them that I never took anything and my son is fine. But they want so badly to do everything they can for their unborn child that they will take anything. Anything."

I asked her whether she had heard of any cases where women were threatened with loss of custody over the issue of AIDS drug compliance, and she recounts the story of a client whose two-year-old daughter was crying so hard whenever it came time to give her the AZT that she stopped giving it to her.

"They found out she wasn't giving it to the child," Guembes says, "and they took her daughter away from her." It took her two years to get her child back, and she was warned that, to keep her, she would have to comply with the medical protocol.

"Now she doesn't miss a dose," Guembes says somberly.

The intimidation experienced by women who test positive for HIV is, in fact, intense. "It's not like with gay men," said Emily Gordon, a social worker and a former health consultant to the New York Department of Health. "With parents, the doctor or social worker will look at the mother and say, 'You love this child? Do you want this child to die?' And she'll walk out with a prescription for whatever the doctor is pushing at that point."

"It's shocking, but nobody cares," agreed Terry McGovern of the HIV Law Project, a group that represents many HIV-positive mothers in their struggles with the system. "It's far from clear that any treatments do any good, and yet these women are viewed as baby killers when they hesitate to give toxic drugs or take them when they're pregnant."

McGovern likens the current battle to the reproductive rights movement. "From a lawyer's viewpoint," she said, "we are squarely within Roe v. Wade territory here, with the big question of whether the mother can overcome the doctor's decision not to take AZT."

For her part, Guembes decided not to take any medication while pregnant or after. (AZT was offered to her years before ACTG 076.) Today, she remains healthy, as does her boy, who is HIV-negative. "When people found out I wanted to have this baby," she recalls, "everybody said that I should have an abortion. Everybody."

That was the informal "standard of care" for all HIV-positive pregnant women in the past—they were counseled to have abortions. Initially, the belief was that 100 percent of babies would inherit their mother's HIV. Even today, women often are told that the risk of transmission with AZT is 50 percent. In fact, it usually takes six to eighteen months for children who are born to HIV-positive mothers but who have not been infected with HIV to revert to negative.

Today Guembes doesn't go around expecting to get sick. "I don't think HIV is the sole cause of AIDS," she says. But her colleagues at the AIDS organization where she works still pressure her relentlessly to start taking medications.

"I just smile at them," she says, "and say, 'Nah, not just yet.'"

What has been said by many people who work with women and HIV is similar to Guembes's story: Growing numbers of mothers are intuitively rejecting the medicines. They often pretend they're taking the drugs and giving them to their children, but in fact they're stockpiling the pills at home, or flushing them down the toilet.

"Mothers will never tell their doctors, but they'll tell me," says Emily Gordon, the New York social worker. "Parents are often very much against using AZT. They feel like they are poisoning their kids."

I asked Ellen Cooper whether she thinks that HIV-positive women's attitudes toward having children are changing. "Probably," she says. "There are some HIV-infected women who are more likely to have children now. But an 8 percent risk of transmission is still a risk. It is different than it was, but it's not zero. An 8 percent risk is a higher risk than most people would take with other congenital diseases. As long as the women understand that, we totally support them if they decide to have a child."

One of the problems with assessing the true toxicity data from 076 is that they are collected in a "Pregnancy Registry," which is largely under the control of the company that makes AZT. But some bits of data have been mined, and they are not exactly reassuring.

AZT was first tested on minority populations in the United States and cohorts of pregnant women in the Third World—the same populations on whom contraceptives are commonly tested. Prior to the launch of 076, data on forty-one women who took AZT during gestation was collected and surveyed by the ACTG OB-GYN Working Group. Two children were born with extra digits on their hands and feet. Other serious birth defects included low-set ears, misshapen craniums, and heart defects. Another study, published the same year as 076 in the *Journal of Acquired Immune Deficiency Syndrome*, studied AZT in pregnant women in India, focusing on birth defects. Out of 104 pregnant women treated with AZT, there were eight reported spontaneous abortions, eight therapeutic abortions, and eight babies (13 percent) born with serious birth defects, including cavities in the chest, abnormal indentations at the base of the spine, misplaced ears, heart problems, extra digits, and albinism. Birth defects generally occur in the population at the rate of 2 to 3 percent of live births. The results of this investigation were described by the study's authors, with what appears now to be some considerable understatement, as "not proving [AZT's] safety" during pregnancy.

Similarly, a 1996 study from the American National Institute of Child Health and Human Development concluded, "In contrast with anecdotal clinical observations and other studies [showing] that Zidovudine favorably influences [fetal] weight-growth rates, our analysis suggests the opposite."

A list of complications caused in animals (rats, mice, dogs, monkeys) subjected to AZT includes: anemia, bone marrow depletion, leukemia, T-cell depletion, atrophy of the thalmus gland, lymphotoxicity, nephrotoxicity, cell death, lung, liver, and vaginal cancer, retarded development, and, worst of all, fetal death.

As a result of such findings, a 1994 study published in the *JAMA* stated categorically that AZT taken during pregnancy resulted in an increased rate of structural birth defects.

"Anecdotally, there certainly have been rumors that some of the HIV-negative children enrolled in 076 have heart problems," says Marion Banzhaf, who works with women and AIDS in New York City as a consultant.

"I agree that it's scary that we do not know what the long-term adverse effects of AZT may be," said Dr. Lynne Mofenson, who co-authored the CDC's recent Perinatal Transmission Treatment recommendations. "But it is clear from the data that the adverse effects so far have been minimal."

"I've never seen any enlarged craniums in the children whose mothers received AZT," says Dr. Cooper, when I questioned her about Kris Chmiel's observation.

"We don't yet know what the long-term effects of AZT may be," she goes on, "but so far we have seen virtually no adverse effects in the short term. The babies are perfectly normal. I have an unpublished paper in front of me that looks at the possibility of tumors developing in these kids. There was not one single tumor. Not one. And no abnormalities either."

"I mean," she adds, "they have cancers, lymphomas, and other problems like that, because cancers tend to be more prevalent in HIV children than in others, but there is no reason to link those cancers to the AZT." Studies, however, have shown that the risk for lymphomas is 70 percent higher in adults who have been on AZT.

"You have to realize," says Nokes, "that they are never going to say that any serious side effect is 'caused' by AZT, because typically, in these children, you can find countless other adverse external factors. Crack. Heroin. Smoking. Alcohol. Hepatitis B and C. So first you would have to reach the high level of complications that is caused by all that, and then exceed that by a wide margin, and then maybe we can start to talk about the adverse effects of AZT."

What also complicates the question is that AIDS, as currently defined by the CDC, is a collection of disparate symptoms in the presence of an HIV antibody. Critics of the almost indiscriminate use of both AZT and other pharmaceuticals have long argued that the drugs used to combat HIV can create some of the very AIDS-related symptoms they are supposed to help ameliorate. Glaxo-Wellcome stated this fact, too, on page 1170 of the *1998 Physician's Desk Reference*: "Serious adverse events have been reported with Retrovir [name brand AZT.... These] pathological changes, similar to that produced by HIV disease, have been associated with prolonged use of Retrovir."

At the National AIDS Malignancy Conference held in Bethesda, Maryland, in 1997, a research paper was presented that acknowledged the positive results of 076 in reducing maternal HIV transmission. "But," the paper continued, "in adult mice, lifetime AZT administration induces vaginal tumors at a 10 to 20 percent incidence." The paper's authors went on to specify that "in female reproductive organs, the controls had no tumors, and there was a 17 percent incidence of ovarian and uterine tumors at the 25 mg dose. Compared to other known chemical carcinogens," the authors concluded, "AZT appears to be a moderately strong transplacental carcinogen"—meaning it's able to cross the placenta.

Critics of the study, most notably Glaxo-Wellcome, insisted that the data was irrelevant, because the researchers had given much higher doses of AZT, proportionally, to their monkey and mice subjects than would be given to humans. The authors, however, insisted that the total drug doses given to the animals were quite similar to those that would be received by any woman who took AZT for about six months. "The data suggest," the researchers concluded, "that the [medical] surveillance of [all] AZT-exposed children should be carried out well into adulthood."

"What's to make us think that there is not going to be some kind of major price to pay somewhere later down the road for giving AZT to these babies?" asks Kathleen Nokes. "And I don't mean a minor price, I mean a major price. All I know is, this drug has been shown to cause vaginal cancer in rodents. It is affecting the blood of these infants, causing various abnormalities. The party line up to this point had been: 'Don't give pregnant women anything'—especially coming off of the big thalidomide study, which everyone in the United States still pats themselves on the back for.

"I don't think we're going to have the answer to the toxicity questions in just a year or two," she continues. "I think we're talking more like six years or, seven, eight, even ten years. A lot of supposed experts are saying, 'Oh come on now, you're overreacting.'"

Nokes does say that she has been reassured somewhat by the fact that AZT is now usually being given in smaller doses and for shorter periods of time than in the years immediately following ACTG 076.

"We don't yet know the long-term effects of AZT or other HIV drugs, that's true," counters Dr. Cooper, "and we are looking very closely at that. But if you compare the terrible risk of contracting HIV, which is always fatal, to the minimal risks of AZT, I would say there is no comparison."

This, then, is precisely where the ideological battle was drawn: To those who were convinced that HIV is "always fatal," AZT, even during pregnancy, was essential. But to those who questioned that presumption, this now-standard treatment for nonsymptomatic and risk-free HIV-positive patients—and their children—came to seem almost diabolical.

It is remembered, if at all, as the "Amsterdam Surprise." A scientific abstract at the 1992 International Conference on AIDS in Amsterdam revealed that a number of clinical AIDS cases exist where doctors could find no trace whatsoever of either HIV-1 or HIV-2.

The mainstream media scrambled to make sense of a startling revelation: There are a significant number of AIDS cases with no trace of HIV. News of the HIV-negative AIDS dominated reports from the Amsterdam conference. It began with a *Newsweek* story, at the start of the conference, describing dozens of cases of classic AIDS—low CD4 cell counts, an immune system indicator, and an array of opportunistic infections—in which the patients continually tested negative for HIV, despite rigorous tests with all of the latest, most sensitive detection technologies. Six of these cases had been reported to Centers for Disease Control and Prevention epidemiologists Thomas J. Spira and Bonnie M. Jones, whose brief abstract catalyzed the media mayhem. Another researcher, Dr. Jeffery Laurence of Cornell Medical College, reported that that he had five patients with classic AIDS symptoms but no HIV. And Luc Montagnier said he had two patients with no HIV detectable in their blood. Dr. David Ho, a researcher in New York, said he had seen eleven HIV-negative cases in New York and California.

On the fourth day of the conference, a California immunologist, Dr. Sudhir Gupta, said he had found a new retrovirus, human intracisternal retrovirus (HICRV), in nine patients who had AIDS but not HIV. Gupta had found the virus in a sixty-six-year-old

California woman who, despite having no risk factors for AIDS and no HIV antibodies, suffered from AIDS-related pneumonia and a low immune-cell count. HICRV was also found in her daughter, then 38, but not in her husband. The daughter had early signs of immune-system dysfunction. The sixty-six-year-old woman had a blood transfusion in 1949 or 1950, before her daughter was born, but Gupta would not speculate as to whether or not she had gotten HICVR from the transfusion. "We can't say if this is a new virus or an old virus," Gupta told the *New York Times*. "All we can say is that it's different from HIV."

Within days of the first report, an ominous atmosphere grew, as more and more scientists stepped up to the microphone in Amsterdam to say that they, too, had seen cases of AIDS with no trace of HIV. By midweek, some thirty cases had been reported and the normally tepid, low-key conference exploded in controversy, despite reassurances from experts that the news was insignificant. Conference participants, journalists, and AIDS activists denounced the CDC for failing to report this phenomenon earlier. Stunned by the outcry, CDC AIDS chief James Curran said: "I don't think it was worth alerting the nation." He and other AIDS researchers were caught flat-footed, not only for failing to explain the phenomenon but also betraying a distressing lack of interest in the cases. Anthony Fauci said at the time that he saw "no reason to panic" over a mere handful of cases, and that it wasn't even known "whether the cases are real." He then did a sudden about face when he realized how much attention the reports were getting. By the third day, he was calling for a special investigation and swearing his team would "get to the bottom of this."

Suddenly, the media was aflood with reports of the cases, making the front pages of the *New York Times, Wall Street Journal,*

USA Today, and other mainstream publications. Spurred by the cases, AIDS made the cover of both *Time* and *Newsweek* simultaneously. CNN started calling HIV "the so-called AIDS virus," and also reported the tiny but illuminating fact that Michael Merson, director of the World Health Organization's Global Program on AIDS, upon learning of the mysterious cases, deleted a reassuring statement that HIV was the cause of AIDS from his opening speech at the conference. The *New York Times* at one point referred to HIV as the virus "thought" to cause AIDS, but, by the second day of the conference, reporting went back to the description of HIV as the "AIDS virus." *Time*, in its cover story, reflected the confusion. "Human immunodeficiency virus (HIV), proclaimed to be the cause of AIDS, has proved a fiendishly fast-moving target, able to mutate its structure to elude detection, drugs, and vaccines. No one knows for sure how HIV destroys the human immune system, and puzzled experts have debated whether the virus is the only culprit at work."

According to the CDC definition of AIDS, a diagnosis can be made only in the presence of HIV antibody. Anyone who tests negative is excluded, not considered an AIDS case, and therefore not included in the general body of AIDS data. And thus, at an Amsterdam press conference, James Curran solved the case of HIV-negative AIDS. He stepped forward and said: "HIV causes AIDS and something else causes the cases reported here today, possibly other viral genes or environmental factors."

In actuality, the existence of HIV-negative AIDS cases was nothing new. Such cases had appeared in the scientific literature for years. But reported as isolated cases, they failed to capture the media's attention. After Amsterdam, the media flocked to speak with Dr. Bijan Safai, who had reported six cases of AIDS with no

HIV at the 1991 International Conference on AIDS in Florence. Safai had been so entirely ignored in Florence that he had decided not to attend the Amsterdam conference. After Safai's presentation in 1991, Robert Gallo jumped up and consumed the question and answer session following Safai's presentation, berating Safai for suggesting that AIDS could exist without the virus Gallo "discovered." After the presentation, only one question besides Gallo's was brought to the floor: "But if a patient dies of *Pneumocystis carinii* pneumonia and had KS and other opportunistic infections," he asked, "but did not have HIV, did that patient die of AIDS or not?" The question was left unanswered.

"They did not want to listen to what I had to say," Safai recalled of the Florence Conference. "Now, suddenly, it's a big story. Everybody in the media is calling me, but nobody was interested last year. It's all so political with AIDS, and I really don't want to get drawn into the politics."

The Amsterdam story also took a strange turn when some papers reported that the new cases must be caused by HIV-3, even though no such strain had been discovered or discussed. "We have only been able to talk about retroviruses since 1980, and there are many others than HIV," noted Dr. Safai, who believes that HIV is the primary—if not the sole cause—of AIDS. "I wouldn't be surprised to see other viruses isolated from people with AIDS. It's very important not to think that there is only this one retrovirus which causes severe immune deficiency and kills people. That's what I was trying to show."

In the end, the CDC invented a new name to label the mysterious cases, thus isolating them from AIDS cases and creating an artificial, if airtight, correlation between HIV and AIDS. The new disease was called "ICL," which stands for idiopathic CD4 lymphocytopenia, which simply means "CD4 cells vanishing for unknown reasons." ICL was described not as HIV-negative AIDS but as a separate, distinct disease grouping, not thought to have one origin, to be caused by a virus, or to be infectious. Compared to HIV-positive AIDS cases, cases of ICL are indeed very rare. But science does not typically measure importance in sheer bulk. Certainly, these cases were no more rare than the first smattering of AIDS cases were in 1981. But they formed an ominous cloud that hangs over AIDS research—one that suggests that immune deficiency is far, far more complicated than previously believed.

Despite their what-me-worry public statements, the U.S. government and the World Health Organization were so concerned about these cases that they launched a major international investigation, held high-level meetings, and even started to design new computer software just to track them. What they were most worried about was the possibility that yet another "deadly virus" was on the loose and was threatening the blood supply. After reassurances that no such threat was evident, the threat died down, and the media moved on. But these cases present an even larger question that continues to haunt certain AIDS researchers: Is there an unknown realm of immune suppression that has nothing to do with HIV? If so, what is the real relationship between HIV and AIDS?

In crime cases, a solid alibi settles everything: Prove you weren't there and you're off the hook. Why not the same for HIV?

The issue of "causation" is one of the most elusive and fractured areas of science. Doctors and researchers have for centuries tried to distinguish the rules by which it is safe to say that a particular organism causes a particular disease. The German bacteriologist Robert Koch is often cited for his four postulates, the first of which is that the accused germ must be present in every case of the disease. But scientists still disagree as to whether Koch's 120-year-old rule can be applied to modern diseases. Still, the place to begin when pinning a germ to a disease is mere detection. You wouldn't diagnosis tuberculosis without a positive TB culture. Nor polio without the polio virus. But with AIDS, all the rules are, apparently, different.

AIDS was given its name when it was still possible to look at it objectively: Acquired Immune Deficiency Syndrome. It was in 1981 that the first cluster of cases were seen in New York and San Francisco, "among previously healthy homosexual men." The defining characteristics were "rare diseases," most notably a skin cancer called Kaposi's sarcoma (KS) and opportunistic infections such as *Pneumocystis carinii* pneumonia (PCP). Researches soon discovered that these men shared an immunological defect—a severe drop in so-called "T-helper" cells, also called CD4 cells. PCP was a real tell-tale sign of immune collapse. It had previously been seen only in patients who were immune-suppressed from cancer or other therapies, or in the very malnourished, such as children in Eastern Europe following World War II. The term AIDS was applied by the CDC, to describe "a disease, at least moderately predictive of a defect in cell-mediated immunity, occurring with no cause for diminished resistance to that disease." HIV and AIDS have been so closely tied as to have become synonymous in the public mind.

But there was never actually a perfect correlation. Only forty percent of the very cases Robert Gallo based his 1984 announcement on were proven to have the virus. The statistic is revealing, because it shows that AIDS researchers were not overly concerned with the correlation issue even then. At long last the

National Institutes of Health offered up the data that spawned the hypothesis in a lengthy 1995 refutation of the argument that HIV might not cause AIDS. Here is the bottom line: In 1984, the NIH isolated HIV in forty-eight of 119 subjects. In San Francisco, HIV was found in people both with and without symptoms of AIDS. Researchers found virus in twenty-seven of fifty-five patients with AIDS and HIV antibodies in 90 percent of 113 people with AIDS.

In other words, from the very beginning it was documented that that fewer than 50 percent of all early-AIDS patients had evidence of true viral infection with HIV. A much higher percentage, close to 90 percent, were antibody positive, but in subsequent years, the HIV-antibody test was deemed flawed, known to produce numerous false-positive results, especially the earliest tests, by cross-reacting with other microbes. CDC epidemiologist Dr. Dawn Smith thinks that the early, poor correlation between HIV and AIDS is an artifact of technology. "The detection techniques used back then to find HIV were not as refined as they are today."

And yet cases of ICL, the disease characterized as AIDS with no HIV, is a topic that is growing and not diminishing on medical databases. In 1993 the World Health Organization reported that its retrospective study, conducted in twenty-one countries, turned up forty-nine cases, as far afield as Zambia, Germany, New Zealand, and Ukraine. A Medline computer search for 1994 yielded thirty-eight entries with case reports; in 1995 there were sixty. A close reading of the literature reveals that ICL cases are still trickling in at a steady pace. Not explosive by any means, but steady.

In the weeks following Amsterdam, the CDC was quick to create a case definition for ICL: 1) Repeated CD4 cell counts below 300 (1,000 is considered normal); 2) Repeated negative blood tests for HIV; and 3) No evidence of immune-suppressive drugs, therapies, or conditions that might explain the immune collapse. They then launched a massive surveillance hunt in an attempt to find all cases. They scanned all of their databases, and alerted all HIV/AIDS clinicians and AIDS researchers in the country to report any cases of HIV-negative immune suppression. Less than three weeks after the Amsterdam conference, the CDC called an emergency meeting in Atlanta, to which more than 270 medical professionals came, including the head of the World Health Organization, Michael Merson.

At the time of the meeting, the CDC was giving the official number of ICL cases as thirty. But by the end of the meeting, a total of 173 cases had in fact been reported by doctors across the country. The questions posed from the outset of the meeting were: Is this a new illness? How common is it? What is the cause or causes? Is the syndrome caused by a transmittable agent? If so, how is it transmitted? And finally: Can it be prevented?

The search for ICL cases went along two main lines: One was a search in the database of AIDS cases to see how many of them were HIV-negative, another was a search among HIV-negative people for low CD4 counts. Of the latter, more than a hundred cases were reported in the meeting, out of several thousand samples. Of the former, a nationwide search of 230,179 AIDS cases yielded 299 who had "AIDS-defining conditions" but were HIV-negative. Of these, investigations were completed on 172, and 134 were "reclassified" after further investigation. Eight were "deceased pediatric patients born of known HIV-positive mothers." In the words of Dr. Martha Rogers of the CDC, "Thirty cases were sero-negative AIDS cases. Two of these thirty cases met the ICL definition."

This raised a tangle of questions: If 299 people had AIDS-defining conditions but tested negative, do they still have AIDS? If there were thirty cases of seronegative AIDS, and HIV is the *cause* of AIDS, then isn't that like saying that water isn't always wet? If the CDC and NIH insist that ICL and AIDS are separate syndromes, clinically and epidemiologically, then why, when ICL cases *are* found to be HIV-positive, do they get reclassified as AIDS? And if two out of thirty seronegative AIDS cases also had ICL, does this mean a person can have both AIDS and ICL? And finally, if 134 people tested negative and then positive, then how reliable is the HIV test?

The CDC has remained resolute that ICL and AIDS are distinct syndromes. In their view, AIDS is caused by HIV and ICL is caused by multiple factors. In a sense, these cases represent a diagnostic crossroads between the orthodox opinions of HIV and skeptical ones, because the take-home message is that HIV is not the *only* cause of AIDS—if by AIDS we mean severe immune suppression. But because AIDS is inextricably bound to HIV in the discourse, there is no language to describe AIDS outside of HIV.

"ICL," some critics contend, is the CDC's semantic creation that attempts to explain the inexplicable simply by naming it. Dr. Smith of the CDC was very forthcoming and did her best to sort out the confusion. "There are clearly ways to become immunosuppressed and ill without being HIV infected," she said. "That's absolutely true. Whether you call that AIDS or not is where we part company." When asked whether there can be AIDS without HIV, she answered: "Well, it depends on what you mean by the term 'AIDS.' That's what makes it complicated." According to Smith, a person can have "AIDS-defining clinical conditions" but still not have AIDS if they lack HIV, and not have ICL (which, when said aloud, rhymes with "pickle") if they have over 330 CD4 cells. "They wouldn't have the *disease* AIDS, because they're not HIV-positive, and they wouldn't have two CD4 counts below the cutoff."

So, what do those people have?

"They just have whatever their condition is," Smith answered, illuminating the occasional madness of modern diagnostic medicine, where numbers, not symptoms, define disease. Many researchers pushed, after hearing news of ICL, for AIDS to be renamed the "HIV disease," which they felt was more specific than AIDS. "If we'd found the virus first," said Smith, "we never would have called anything AIDS. What we use AIDS to mean clinically is severe immmnodepression due to HIV infection."

"So," I offer, "as far as the CDC is concerned, AIDS can exist only with HIV infection."

"Right," replied Smith.

The CDC's Dr. Spira stressed that ICL is clinically distinct from AIDS, primarily in that the immune decline is not usually progressive, although it is persistent, and that some of the immunological parameters are different in ICL and AIDS. But reading through all the reports, the picture that emerges about ICL is essentially this: The patient has illnesses indicative of a failed immune system. Their T-cells are tested and often found to be extremely low, for no apparent reason. Some die, others don't. That fits the CDC's first definition of AIDS perfectly: "a disease at least moderately predicative of a defect in cell-mediated immunity, occurring with no known cause for diminished resistance to that disease."

There is no question that these cases would have been diagnosed as AIDS had they tested positive for HIV, a fact confirmed by Spira. Compounding the confusion is that the

AIDS definition has undergone countless changes. It has been progressively broadened over the years to encompass more and more symptoms. (You can't have AIDS if you have fewer than 200 CD4 cells, and one of the "AIDS indicator diseases," and an HIV-positive test result.) And now there is a new category: Those who qualify neither for AIDS or ICL. When the CDC scanned its AIDS databases—these are people who have already been diagnosed with AIDS—they found 299 who did not have HIV. And yet, only a fraction of those fit the ICL definition. How are the remaining HIV-negative AIDS cases classified?

"There is no official category called HIV-negative AIDS," Smith replied, confirming the problem that if they are not counted, they do not exist, which skews the correlation data that the HIV question hinges on.

"Many more cases of ICL were initially reported than are in the CDC's records," recalls AIDS researcher Robert Root-Bernstein, author of *Rethinking AIDS: The Cost of Premature Consensus,* "because of the way they ended up defining it. It's a very strict definition, much stricter than AIDS. My recollection is that there were between 400 and 600 cases of HIV-negative AIDS initially, but most of them were thrown out as not ICL."

AIDS, by contrast, suffers the opposite problem—the numbers get inflated as the definition broadens each year.

"The big shock for me was to discover that there is a whole other category of people who get no diagnosis at all," noted Root-Bernstein. "They die without a diagnosis." Root-Bernstein recalls a medical-school colleague who told him about the case of his father, who had traveled around the world, and wound up of dying of something that "looked like AIDS." But he didn't have

HIV, so he wasn't an AIDS case. He didn't have below 300 CD4 cells, so he didn't have ICL: "My friend said his father died with no diagnosis.... I suspect the problem is bigger than we think it is, but not as huge as AIDS."

"You mean HIV-positive AIDS?" I ask.

"Sorry. Yes."

In 1993, *BioTechnology* published a paper by Peter Duesberg in which Duesberg attacked the medical establishment's claim of overwhelming correlation between HIV and AIDS. Duesberg cited many weak spots, among them that the CDC does not actually document HIV tests along with HIV diagnosis. This correlates with the point made by many AIDS doctors and community representatives that many people refuse to take an HIV test, for fear of losing insurance or employment, or for fear of social stigma. Hence, their AIDS diagnoses are made in the absence of a test.

Duesberg pointed out in his paper that the CDC's director of the HIV/AIDS division, Harold Jaffe, acknowledged in 1993 that the HIV status of 43,606 out of the 253,448 recorded AIDS cases in the U.S. was "not tested." Duesberg then added the 10,360 cases diagnosed before the test was instituted. Citing data from the CDC's Technical Information Activity, he added up "not tested" AIDS—cases from 1986 through 1992—and arrived at 62,272 AIDS cases for whom HIV status was never known, a so-called "presumptive diagnosis." That's 18,666 more than Jaffe reported.

Duesberg went on to cite 4,621 cases of demonstrably HIV-free immunodeficiency, which he claims are documented in the U.S., Europe, and Africa using the clinical AIDS definition. Jaffe, at the time of Duesberg's writing, put the figure at eighty-nine.

Duesberg included three staggering stats: Out of a cohort of 4,383 African AIDS cases from the Ivory Coast, Zambia, and Zaire, more than half—2,215—were found to be HIV-negative when tested. Out of 227 AIDS cases in Ghana, 135—or 59 percent—were found to be HIV-negative.

In 1996, I interviewed Judith Lopez, who suffered from debilitating immune deficiency beginning in 1970, when she was thirty-years-old. "I got sick a decade before AIDS existed, so I think it's safe to assume I'm negative," she said. Lopez had the symptoms of what was later called Chronic Fatigue Syndrome, which shares many symptoms with AIDS. In fact, some researchers believe that the two syndromes are related. In 1988 Lopez, who had no risk factors for AIDS, collapsed at work, went to bed, and stayed there for the next five years. She was allergic to almost everything, including paper—which prevented her from reading. "One day I opened my mouth," she recalled. "It was totally covered with candidiasis, which was hanging in strings like a fern. My immune system had been totally destroyed."

Lopez felt she had all the symptoms that are also attributed to AIDS. "I had candidiasis, dementia, muscle atrophy, wasting. I weighed eighty pounds. I certainly looked like an AIDS patient. When I go down the list, the only thing I lacked was a positive test."

"The big issue here," said Root-Bernstein, "is whether there's a single cause for all immune deficiencies or whether there are multiple causes for immune deficiencies. We don't know whether AIDS is a single category, much less whether ICL is a single category, or whether both are supercategories to something much larger.... These cases illustrate that immune suppression can occur without HIV. Well, if that is so, then it follows logically that the same immune suppression, independent of HIV, could also be at work with HIV present. Maybe HIV is doing nothing. There is certainly a wealth of knowledge and insight to be found in these negative cases."

Sadly, however, almost all researchers working with ICL said that the whole endeavor was called off in the mid-'90s for lack of interest. Frequently cited was that there were so few cases, compared with HIV-positive AIDS cases.

"As soon as they realized that there was no new retrovirus at work, they basically moved on," said Jean Druckmiller, AIDS surveillance coordinator of the Wisconsin Bureau of Public Health. "I haven't heard anything about this in a long time."

According to the 268-page transcript of the 1992 CDC meeting, not one word was uttered that drew into question the relationship between HIV and AIDS. One doctor tried to say that rather than focus on viral causes for everything, they should be looking at non-viral co-factors, but he was cut off and told that time was limited. He was the only speaker at the entire conference who was cut off.

Howard Temin, the late Nobel Laureate who discovered reverse transcriptase, the hallmark of retroviruses, spoke toward the end of the meeting and articulated the zeitgeist with his reassuring words. "We have heard of some cases that meet the definition of [of AIDS]," Temin said, "and did not have demonstrable HIV. This would not mean that HIV does not cause AIDS. I don't think anyone on the panel here does not accept that the great majority of what is called AIDS is caused by HIV. There may be 200,000 or 300,000 such cases, and there are thirty of these other things. It merely means that we should again change the definition so that there will be HIV-positive AIDS and HIV-negative AIDS."

"But none of what is presented here," Temin promised, "at all affects the previous conclusion of the majority of scientists in this area, that HIV causes AIDS in the sense of the major pandemic that's ravaging the world."

"If the spread of AIDS continues at this rate, in 1996 there could be one billion people infected; five years later, hypothetically ten billion people; however, the population of the world is only five billion. Could we be facing the threat of extinction during our lifetime? Even before our children are grown?"

Theresa Crenshaw, President's AIDS Commission, 1987

HIV tests detect footprints, never the animal itself. These footprints, antibodies, are identified by means of molecular protein weights, and were limited to two in 1984, when the first test was developed and patented, but over the years expanded to include many proteins previously not associated with HIV. A majority of HIV-positive tests, when retested, come back indeterminate or negative. In many cases, different results emerge from the same blood tested in different labs. There are currently at least eleven different criteria for how many and what proteins—expressed in "band density"—signal "positive." The most stringent criteria (four bands) are upheld in Australia and France; the least stringent (two bands), in Africa, where an HIV test is not even required as a part of an AIDS diagnosis. The U.S. standard is three reactive bands. It has been pointed out that a person could revert to being HIV-negative simply by buying a plane ticket from Uganda to Australia.

UNAIDS, the Joint United Nations Programme on HIV/AIDS, estimates that, as of the end of 2004, 39.4 million people worldwide are living with "HIV/AIDS." But this number is derived from a statistical range, wherein UNAIDS estimates that the true number might be anywhere between 35.9 and 44.3 million people. These Projections of the epidemic, however, are not based on death statistics. Rather, they are based on estimates of HIV "infection," estimates that are themselves inferred from projections of HIV-positive blood samples. The UNAIDS statistics therefore represent the organization's estimate of the number of people *presumed* to be

infected with HIV—people who would test positive for the HIV
blood test—and thus be "living with HIV/AIDS." (Estimates of the
number of clinical AIDS cases worldwide have also been expanding
exponentially. Between 1994 and 1995, the World Bank—working
from World Health Organization statistics—documents a ten-fold
increase in AIDS cases. It is a baffling change. In 1994, 152,911
AIDS cases were reported to the WHO; by 1995, the World Bank
documents that some think that this number might have grown to
1.8 million. See Appendix I.) Africa, as the media never tires of
telling us, has become ground zero of the AIDS epidemic.

But the figures we are always given for HIV sero-prevalance in
Africa are based on sample studies taken at a few select pre-natal
clinics. I cannot reproduce all of them here, because the figures
are like billowing cloud formations: Always very big, very round
figures, always "estimates," and always capped with a line like
"Experts say the real figure could be three times that high," which
means that they are arbitrarily arrived at in the first place.

I once spoke to a UNAIDS official in a casual setting—he was
sitting at a bar and we struck up a conversation. "Not to insult to
you," I said, "but the figures your organization puts out are pure
fiction."

"Pure fiction," he confirmed, leaning against the bar with
his elbow.

"Why then, do you put them out?"

"Money," he said. "It's all about fundraising. High figures
bring in money."

When you get such officials face to face, caught off guard,
they tend to tell you the truth, in simple language.

Most sub-Saharan African nations don't even keep death
statistics, which could be used to check the ever-billowing HIV

"estimates" against. Instead, there is a climate of shame attached to the question itself—the question of whether there is *any* relationship between UNAIDS HIV/AIDS statistics and a syndrome of infectious immune suppression that is *new,* and separate from other tropical diseases which it mimics exactly. Rian Malan, the South African writer, has been wrestling with the African AIDS figures since *Rolling Stone* assigned him to write a story reaffirming President Mbeki's venality—for "ignoring" AIDS in South Africa—in 2000. Malan spent a year trying to shore up the official story, the official figures, in order to show how wrong Mbeki was for questioning it. But Malan came back to the magazine on the opposite end of his own premise. Mbeki, it turned out, had a point. The figures are all generated by computer models, large AIDS programs, and the like. Malan set out in search of physical proof of AIDS—a new illness that was striking down sexually active people in their prime—in South Africa. He was not even able to find an increase in overall death statistics in South Africa. Finally, in desperation, he tried to find the bodies, so to speak. He traced coffin sales and interviewed coffin builders. He found that they were idle, selling next to nothing, and were worried about going out of business.

Malan's mother begged him to drop the story. "Shut up," she said. "They'll put you in a straightjacket."

He was attacked in the South African media. He never did find it—the AIDS epidemic in South Africa. One can always find sick and old dying people, but Malan looked for AIDS, as something truly distinguishable from common tropical diseases.

Instead, if you really study it, you find that AIDS in Africa is a communal projection based on estimates of HIV-positives, culled from select and small samples, which in turn are doubled, tripled, even quadrupled, then pumped out via the WHO and its satellite organizations to the world's news organizations, who reprint the figures dutifully and unquestioningly. No differentiation is made between HIV-positive antibodies, disease, and death.

As Drs. David Rasnick and Christian Fiala reported in their 2003 paper "But—What About Africa?" (submitted to the *British Medical Journal* but rejected) far from being "wiped off the map," the population on the continent of Africa exploded during the very period of time it was supposedly being decimated by AIDS. It went from 378 million people in 1980 to 652 million in 2000. It grew by 274 million people—about the size of the entire U.S. population.

Tom Bethell reported this fact and others in the *American Spectator* in 2005, adding that mainstream media outlets, including the *New York Times,* have oversimplified infection rates in Africa, never reporting problems, "conditions that trigger false positives," or lack of widespread testing. Still, the attitude prevails that to question the figures about AIDS in Africa is to be an AIDS "denialist," which is, of course, intended to update the sinister figure of the Holocaust denier. You are not trying to be accurate, or examine epidemiology, or make sure diseases don't all become conflated into one huge clump labeled AIDS—you are instead denying mass death, denying what is known to every school child. It is as though a message of imminent mass death, from sex no less, is a kind of humanitarian courtesy to the continent of Africa.

I've traveled to Africa many times—east, central, west, north, and south—in search of my own answers. One particular story sticks in my mind and bears repeating. I was in the Rakai district of Uganda and came upon a village.

A man walked over to greet me, clasping my hand. Because I am white, he immediately assumed I was there on behalf of a Western

AIDS group and that I was going to preach the importance of condom use. Holding my hand in his, he said imploringly: "Madam, let me tell you something about us. We *must* procreate."

The advice to "use a condom every time" in rural Uganda is clearly absurd, considering how many children they bear, and how many die in infancy. Embarrassed, I assured him I was not there to preach condom use, but to ask some questions about AIDS.

"Terrible," he said, shaking his head. "I have had two brothers and one sister die of AIDS already."

"I'm sorry," I said. "What did they die of?"

"*Slim.* AIDS."

"I mean what was the cause of death?"

"Ahh. Well, my brother for instance, he had malaria and we couldn't afford to get him treatment, so he died."

"So he died of untreated malaria," I said.

"Yes, malaria."

"Why did you say he died of AIDS?"

He shrugged. "*Slim*, AIDS... is a formula for everything here. When somebody dies we call it *slim*."

The WHO had allotted $6 million for AIDS for 1992-93, around the time I was there. All other infectious diseases combined, barring TB, received only $57,000. Perhaps it is no wonder that health care workers there have learned to "call everything AIDS."

The clinical definition of AIDS in Africa is stunningly broad and generic, designed to mean just about anything and nothing. It is in no way comparable to western definitions. It's called the "Bangui definition" of AIDS, because it was established in the city of Bangui in the Central African Republic, at a conference in 1985. The definition requires neither a positive HIV test nor a T-cell count, as in the West, but only the presence of chronic diarrhea, fever, significant weight loss, and asthenia, as well as other minor symptoms. These are also the symptoms of most non-AIDS diseases, including malnutrition, malaria, and parasitic infections, in Africa. In 1994 Bangui was finally updated to suggest the use of an HIV test, but in practice, they are prohibitively expensive.

The reality is that, in Africa, estimates of the HIV-positive population are estimated using the results from a limited number of HIV tests. But as many critics have tried, in vain, to point out, this is another reason why the projected picture is so utterly distorted: the HIV test itself is unreliable.

A group of researchers based in Perth Australia, headed by the nuclear physicist Eleni Eleopolis-Papadopoulis, have for years been publishing blistering, detailed critiques on the very interface between AIDS projections and AIDS realities. Their main target is the HIV test—and the Western Blot test in particular—which they say is the very gateway to a series of Escher-like stairways of presumptions leading nowhere except to each other. The so-called "Perth Group" has argued in several meticulously documented papers, read and studied chiefly by so-called AIDS dissidents, that HIV is not a coherent, gold-standardized, *purified* retroviral entity, but rather a series of proteins which are not unique constituents of HIV, and can appear wherever certain immune stressors, microbes, and antigens congregate at high concentrations. Eleopolis-Papadopolis and her colleague Dr. Valendar Turner, an Oxford educated heart surgeon at the Royal Perth Hospital, have documented up to seventy proteins that can cause a false positive result on a Western Blot test, including those for malaria, TB, and even pregnancy itself. HIV is not an "it" in the way that we imagine it—unlike other viral infections, it is extremely hard to test for because, as Peter Duesberg has pointed out, "it's barely there"—it can only be detected with generously broad antibody tests and highly sensitive DNA tests, like PCR, which can find a needle in a haystack.

HIV was never isolated in a way that would have provided a so-called Gold Standard to test for its presence or absence. From the outset, it was inferred by laboratory identifications. If you have this, this, and this protein, it *means* HIV, on the theory that those protein combinations are unique to HIV and not found elsewhere. It is like the difference between footprints of a tiger and the tiger itself. If you see the footprints, you assume the tiger has passed through. But what if the footprints, as the Perth Group has argued, are not those of a tiger? Their research has shown that the proteins said to be unique to HIV, and which signal HIV on the antibody test, are not at all unique to HIV.

The two proteins considered most specific to and indicative of HIV's presence are p24 and p41. (Written as such because the proteins correspond to a particular molecular weight.) In the early years of AIDS, a number of people were told they were infected with HIV based *only* on the presence of p24 or p41. The U.S. Multicenter AIDS Cohort Study (MACS), began in the early 1980s, testing and studying 5,000 gay men. All of them were told they were HIV-positive, and presumably most of them began taking AIDS drugs. One band was considered sufficient proof of HIV infection in the United States until 1990. One third of people transfused with HIV-free blood later developed antibodies to p24. Fifty percent of 144 dogs tested for HIV in 1990 were found to have antibodies to one or more HIV proteins.

In 1988, the U.S. Army tested over a million soldiers with the ELISA AIDS test and found 12,000 were positive. Half were negative on a repeat ELISA. Two thirds failed to react on a first

Western Blot test, and some of those failed to react on a repeat Western Blot. The point is that all 12,000 would have been called "HIV infected" in Africa but very few would have been called that in the West.

In another disturbing study, HIV-free mice tested positive for HIV when they were injected with cells from other HIV-free mice.

One quarter of HIV-free blood donors in the West were found to have reactive bands on the HIV Western Blot test. The HIV Reference Laboratory admitted to Turner and Eleopoulis, when pressed, that these were caused by cross-reacting non-HIV antibodies. In a 1997 interview in the now defunct AIDS journal *Continuum*, Turner explained: "Now, the way you get your cross-reacting, non-HIV induced antibodies is to give your immune system a few belts. And the more belts, and the more closely spaced, the more likely a person tested will have cross reacting antibodies. But we know in places like Africa this kind of thing is happening all the time. And it happens across all the AIDS risk groups. The very people you're testing for HIV are those with the greatest chance of non-specifically induced antibodies. So we have this grotesque paradox. One quarter of pristine, well-fed Australian blood donors have one or more HIV Western Blot bands, and that might include four bands, but they're not infected with HIV. But in Africa, poverty stricken, malnourished, Ugandan subsistence farmers with malaria or tuberculosis, or repeated attacks of dysentery, have buckets of cross reacting antibodies but if they've got just two bands on the Western Blot, not four, they *are* infected with HIV. Do you know anyone who can explain this?"

Whether or not people ought to submit to taking an "AIDS test" has long been the subject of furious debate. The impact on the life or lives of the people who do take the test—if it comes back positive—is incalculable, since HIV is still largely associated with surefire death. The debate about the HIV antibody test has been long, complex, and anguished. No single diagnostic test in the history of modern medicine has had such a momentous impact on the lives of the individuals who rely on it. Since the beginning of the AIDS crisis, people have had very dramatic reactions to receiving positive test results—lapsing into chronic depression and anxiety, quitting, or losing their jobs, taking very toxic medications, getting divorced, having abortions, taking their lives and sometimes even other people's lives—all based, not on diagnosis of AIDS, but merely a positive antibody test. Given that the test holds such power, its flaws and shortcomings are extremely significant. Unfortunately, it is only since the early '90s that this immensely important subject has been investigated.

In addition to the Perth group's critique of the Western Blot test, significant criticisms have also been directed at the ELISA, which was the first test developed for HIV in 1985, developed specificly to screen out HIV from the blood supply. The test is highly sensitive and very nonspecific, which means it gives a positive result easily even when there is no HIV present. At one time, as many as four out of five ELISA tests could not be confirmed by the Western Blot.

One of the most important problems with overstating HIV infection in Africa is that overestimation muddles the reality of the epidemic in other parts of the world. At the dawn of the AIDS epidemic, doomsday figures were announced for the U.S. and the world—some held out the possibility of human extinction. But, as Valendar Turner notes, the African AIDS "epidemic," no matter its supposed magnitude, is useless in predicting the spread of the disease elsewhere, especially in the West. "Under such diagnostic rigor," Turner writes about assumptions of HIV infection in Africa, "the example of thousands of African men and women, who are essentially suffering from symptoms and diseases all called other names before 1981, is held up as proof that the West is menaced by the threat of heterosexually transmitted AIDS."

Turner is referring to the by now discarded notion—on the scrapheap of so many discarded AIDS fictions—that an unchecked AIDS epidemic in the West can be predicted by the African epidemic, where "AIDS," as we were relentlessly told, "spreads heterosexually." The long and complicated history of the AIDS epidemic in the U.S., however, shows that this is a supremely misguided notion. Indeed, the first heterosexual AIDS epidemic predicted for the U.S. simply never happened. That a heterosexual AIDS epidemic was ever predicted in the West is simply never mentioned anymore, rather like Y2K.

A vast array of epidemiological indicators came to light during the '90s during investigations of the threat posed by heterosexual transmission of AIDS. In 1991, a study published in the medical journal *Fertility and Sterility* addressed a very basic question: Can HIV be found in the semen of HIV-positive men? The results were deeply perplexing. Semen samples of twenty-five HIV-positive men were studied, and it was discovered that only four showed any trace of HIV. While epidemiological reports indicate quite clearly that AIDS is spread two ways—through blood and semen—the findings placed considerable doubt on the role HIV plays in relation to the spread of the disease. The authors of the study acknowledged, in a rather understated way, that "very little information exists regarding [HIV's] prevalence in semen and mechanisms underlying its sexual transmission."

The semen samples were taken from people both with and without AIDS and were tested with what was then brand new polymerase chain reaction (PCR) technology, which measured the presence of virus in semen far more accurately than previous methods had. Amazingly, however, similar information about HIV and semen had been available almost since HIV was first isolated in 1984. Early on Robert Gallo published a paper stating that he had found HIV in the semen of two AIDS patients, but curiously, Gallo failed to mention how many patients he had studied and not found HIV in. "We don't know how many people he looked for HIV in. He simply reported that he found it in two," observed Dr. Robert Root-Bernstein, who spent several years scrutinizing Gallo's HIV-AIDS data. "In terms of peer review," he said, "it failed utterly and miserably. It's hard to believe what kind of non-science they got away with."

Another study, reported around the same time as Gallo's, examined the semen of twelve AIDS patients and found HIV in only one. Yet this seemingly startling observation went largely unnoticed and undiscussed for years. "Those first two papers were the only ones around on HIV in semen for several years, and they were very misleading," remembers Root-Bernstein. "They made it seem like, 'Well, we looked at these people and clearly HIV is present in the semen and so AIDS can be transmitted by way of semen.' And that's how it was left. The fact is, we still do not know how AIDS is transmitted."

From 1986 through 1988, several more studies were done on HIV in semen, using more accurate testing methods. "What they found," says Root-Bernstein, "was that between 25 and 30 percent of the AIDS patients they looked at had HIV in their semen. But if you read the papers carefully, it turns out they're talking about one to ten 'copies' per ejaculate, or one copy of virus per million units of sperm, which isn't enough to spread an infection. HIV is present to that degree in salvia, breast milk, vaginal fluid—and those are not modes of transmission. You generally need thousands or millions of copies of any virus for it to be infective."

This data raised questions about HIV's infectivity, especially by means of heterosexual sex. The very question is so taboo that one hesitates to ask it: How does HIV transmit, if it's not in semen? Dr. Michael Lange, an infectious disease specialist at St. Luke's-Roosevelt Hospital in New York City, believes that AIDS is transmitted sexually, but is skeptical of HIV's role in the transmission of the disease. "I think there's definitely an infectious agent at work here.... I'm not entirely convinced that it's HIV, or that it's one agent—it could be a combination. But certainly AIDS is infectious."

"I've heard," Root-Bernstein told me in 1992, "that they're pretty concerned about this over at the NIH. I would be, too, if I were them." In the early '90s, after two workshops on HIV transmission, NIH researchers dismissed the 1991 semen studies as not "significant." They claimed that a 1992 study found HIV in the semen of twenty-eight out of twenty-eight studied. But the study, published by the *Journal of Acquired Immune Deficiency Syndromes*, confirms the 1991 data, if you look closely enough. HIV was not found in twenty-eight out of twenty-eight, but rather HIV antibodies were found in only seven of the twenty-eight, which reflects the 25 percent figure found in earlier studies.

Even in patients with full-blown AIDS, HIV is often hard to locate. Studies of AIDS patients have shown, since HIV was isolated in 1984, that only 50 percent of them have evidence of the virus itself, while 90 percent have antibodies. A good percentage of those who are HIV-positive may not actually have the virus.

A study done by AIDS researcher Dr. Nancy Padian followed 175 discordant couples—one positive, one negative—who all had unprotected sex for ten years, to see at what rate HIV would transmit. There was not one transmission. Padian concluded, illogically but diplomatically, that it "takes on average 1,000 unprotected sexual encounters for HIV to transmit." Most people don't have anywhere near that many sexual encounters in their lifetimes.

But confusingly, there have also been cases in which people swear they've gotten AIDS from one single sexual act. Alison Gertz, for instance, the young, affluent heterosexual woman who said she caught AIDS from a man she slept with once, graced many magazine covers across the country in 1989. Suddenly, the media were making a tremendous deal out of what was in reality a very rare example, while insisting that the cases like it were the wave of the future. Although the media favor the dramatic, terror-ridden, Russian roulette model of HIV-AIDS transmission, such cases do not reflect the scientific facts.

How HIV is or isn't spreading has been one of the most inflammatory points of the entire AIDS debate. But by now it seems clear that the "explosion" of heterosexual AIDS is a no-show.

Regardless of how many HIV-positive people there are, the number of potential cases of AIDS in the heterosexual community appears to be self-limiting, because unlike most sexually transmitted diseases, AIDS does not transmit easily in both directions between males and females, therefore inhibiting heterosexual spread. For example, adult cases of AIDS in New York City in 1990 as a result of female-to-male transmission totaled one. In 1991, there were none. From 1981 to 1992, when there were 30,943 men with AIDS in New York, there were, in total, only twelve documented cases of female-to-male transmission; in 1993, the New York City

Health Department changed their method of gathering statistics about heterosexual infection, making such information almost impossible to gather today.

The question of the heterosexual AIDS explosion has been volleyed back and forth between the two opposing camps—those who say it will happen and those who say it won't—for years, unresolved despite a conclusive body of data that shows AIDS is not erupting among heterosexuals. The vast campaign to convince the heterosexual community that "AIDS does not discriminate" is turning out to be politically correct but factually bankrupt AIDS-speak. Twenty-five years after the first AIDS cases appeared, it still remains contained, for the most part, among the initial risk groups.

Dr. Joseph Sonnabend walked out on the organization he had founded, The American Foundation for AIDS Research (AmFAR), primarily because he refused to participate in what he saw as the fraudulent terror campaign. "The AIDS Medical Foundation was sending out this press release saying that nobody is safe, everybody is going to get it—and all that," he recalled. "When I heard this, I totally freaked out. It was all just nonsense. I called them up and said, 'Do you know what's going to happen as a result of what you are doing? You're going to freak out heterosexual men, you're going to destroy relationships, marriages. And another thing, you're going to promote violence against gay men. People are going to say this thing is a plague and it's coming from gay men, and they're going to beat them up at random.' All of which has come true."

At the time, however, AmFAR's then-public relation director, Terry Beirn, who has since died of AIDS, was not about to let Sonnabend or anybody else get in the way of the fund-raising that was just getting into full swing. "I couldn't fight Terry,"

Sonnabend recalled. "He was very determined. It was pretty clear already then that AIDS was not a significant threat to heterosexuals. He knew that this heterosexual AIDS thing was a hoax, but he said he had to do it to raise money. And certainly, you could argue that unless those heterosexual male politicians in Washington thought that sex could kill, they weren't going to release any money. But my response to that was, if you raise money on a false premise, that money's going to be put to no good. And in fact, that's exactly what happened. The money was raised to protect heterosexual men from a disease they're not going to get anyway. So what have these hundreds of millions of research dollars given us? Nothing. AIDS education? All I see is terror and confusion.... But on the other hand, I can see the value in supporting this notion of spread, primarily in order to protect women.... Because women are getting AIDS from men, but men are not getting AIDS from women. And men will only wear condoms if they think they themselves are at risk."

"The only interesting thing about any disease is how to control it," noted British epidemiologist Gordon Stewart in 1992. He had been asked by the World Health Organization to write a report on social and behavioral factors in communicable diseases, including AIDS, in 1983. Stewart, emeritus professor of public health at the University of Glasgow, made statistical projections of AIDS for several years. His projections were based on what the pattern of spread has been—not what it might be in an imagined worst-case scenario. While projections made by the WHO and other health organizations have been grossly exaggerated from what has actually come to pass by tens and sometimes hundreds of thousands, Stewart's have been uncannily precise, sometimes off by just a few cases. "Nobody wants to look at the facts about this disease," said

Stewart. "It's the most extraordinary thing I've ever seen. I've sent countless letters to medical journals pointing out the epidemiological discrepancies and they simply ignore them. The fact is, this whole heterosexual AIDS thing is a hoax."

Female prostitutes, the most obvious risk group for any STD, are baffling AIDS researchers. Among American prostitutes, HIV is not spreading, despite studies showing that most of them do not generally use condoms. And even if they had begun to use condoms in recent years, surely cases should have been cropping up from the years before there was awareness about AIDS. But all the studies with prostitutes conclude the same thing: HIV is primarily found among prostitutes who are also IV-drug users. In 1996, 83 percent of American AIDS cases were either gay or IV-drug users.

On May 1, 1996, the *Wall Street Journal* confirmed this in a front-page story, "Health Hazard: AIDS Fight is Skewed by Federal Campaign Exaggerating Risks," which reported that AIDS, as the CDC had defined it, was virtually nonexistent among heterosexuals with no risk factors for HIV. Coauthored by Atlanta bureau chief Amanda Bennett and staff writer Anita Sharpe, the article was the result of a yearlong investigation, which concluded that "for most heterosexuals, the risk from a single act of sex [is] smaller than ever getting hit by lightening. In the U.S., the disease was, and remains, largely the scourge of gay men, their sex partners, and new born children." "The general impression out there about heterosexual spread," the *Wall Street Journal*'s Bennett later told me, "was not buttressed by the facts. We're not saying that heterosexual transmission is a myth. There is heterosexual transmission. There is some risk to everyone.... [F]rom a public health perspective, the risk is so much greater to people in disenfranchised groups. The impression that there is a huge heterosexual risk to everyone has had the effect of steering the focus away from where the problem is."

Oprah Winfrey predicted in 1987 that "one in five heterosexuals could be dead from AIDS at the end of the next three years."

Indeed, fear mongering, including that propagated by AmFAR, was rampant in the early years of the epidemic.

But while nobody was really paying attention, in a single extraordinary sleight of hand, everything that could not be explained about the predicted heterosexual epidemic in the United States, or in any other Western nation, found a convenient and faraway continent where few could ever check their claims against reality. Losing none of their piety or implicit guilt, and undeterred by the abysmal failure of their hypothesis about the level of HIV infection to live up to a single one of the predictions made for it, many believers had a new kind of pepper spray to stop any critical thinker in his or her tracks. It consisted of four words: "Well, *what about Africa?*"

With this question the whole thing simply imploded into an incoherent and startlingly racist bouillabaisse of pseudo-science. *What about Africa?* Africans were managing to spread the reluctant retrovirus like "wildfire," the media reported, precisely along the lines of the failed heterosexual "epidemic" in the West. It was proof, almost everyone agreed, that AIDS could indeed spread rampantly through heterosexual sex. But how was it possible for AIDS to spread among heterosexuals in Africa, when, in the U.S., no such epidemic had occurred?

The theories were, from the outset, breathtakingly unfounded and insulting—that African men like their women "dry," and even force them to jam wads of drying herbs and spices up their vaginas (as reported by Mark Schoofs in the *Village Voice*, work that was awarded the Pulitzer Prize), that African men routinely rape child virgins because of their belief that this might cure AIDS, that African men enjoy "rough sex," which causes nicks and scrapes, allowing points of entrée for the virus that you don't get in the Western world. The best that can be said of these recent myths about HIV's spread in Africa is that they are a slight improvement over even more racist ideas about how HIV "originated" in Africa, and of the early myths about spread. These were openly discussed in medical journals by top AIDS researchers in the 1980s, and included claims such as that AIDS spread through Africa by way of people having sex with monkeys, engaging in extreme sexual promiscuity, blood drinking rituals, and allowing children to play with dead monkeys.

You can say just about anything about AIDS in Africa without raising eyebrows—except of course, that the statistics are fictional and the disease widely mislabeled. You also cannot say that the antibody test is inaccurate or that the drugs being pressed upon the people there may be harmful. The entire epidemiological premise of a heterosexual African AIDS epidemic rests on variations of a single theme rooted in ancient Anglican fears, rendered appropriate in the age of AIDS anxiety, now AIDS-in-Africa anxiety: That African sexuality is fundamentally *different* from Western sexuality. Rougher. Drier.

If you ask a person who adheres to the mainstream apocalypse model of AIDS in Africa just what *kind* of sex Africans are having that they are spreading HIV like wildfire, they will generally answer: "Dry sex."

You can either drop it, or you can ask them to follow the logic all the way through. "Dry sex. That means sex where the woman has either taken great pains to dry herself out, while rearing perhaps ten children and struggling to feed them all, or, it means sex that is 'dry' because the woman is utterly unwilling and repelled by the man. In which case the word is *rape*. Are we to believe that most sex on the continent of Africa is involuntary, on the part of the woman?"

"AIDS ideology is essentially racist," says Anthony Brink—a South African lawyer who has written three books documenting the battle so far between the AIDS drugs-into-South-Africa activists and the Mbeki-led resistance, to which Brink is central, having provided the government with comprehensive documentation for the toxicities and flawed science of the two main AIDS drugs pushed there—AZT and nevirapine.

Mbeki has been routinely savaged in the almost all-white South African press for questioning the wisdom of pressing acutely toxic, unproven AIDS drugs onto malnourished, already sickly black South Africans, since the "controversy" exploded in 1999. He has been universally pilloried, in the U.S. media as well. Brink sees racism where others see benevolent concern. "It's so poisonous," Brink noted, on the phone from his home in Cape Town. "It's so *metaphysically* poisonous. In this country, we've just come through a racist, fascist dictatorship involving white supremacism and *untermenschen*, and AIDS ideology provides a whole new framework for those ancient racist ideas to bubble back up. It was accepted by gay men so widely because of non-acceptance of their being, and it's been sold to black people for the same reason. It taps into feelings of inferiority. And it draws on ancient racial antipathy and loathing. It permeates all AIDS-thinking. It's like, 'Oh you bestial people, you can't control yourselves and now you're paying the holy price. If you listen to these AIDS researchers speak, they *say* it. We have a professor of HIV/AIDS research here named Gerry Cordavia, from Durban University Medical School, and he speaks about the 'unbridled sexuality of newly-liberated people.' Can you fucking believe it? This is what he says caused AIDS to *rip* through our country. Unbelievable. And another one, professor Cameron Hume, he says things like: 'The problem with AIDS in our country calls for a *tough, aggressive* approach.' Except for Mandela and a few other holy-rollers, AIDS is largely a white-driven paranoia, no question about it. Blacks don't buy it.

"Mbeki always highlights this in his speeches—these sexual stereotypes, these apocryphal kind of urban legend-type stories about African men liking their women dry, and the women drying themselves out with herbs and spices or whatever, to oblige their men. All this unbelievable rubbish. The men completely out of control and the women as victims. Listen, we come from an apartheid past, so white people don't really know black people in this country. And sure, it's getting better, but in Cape Town, the suburbs are lilly-white, and I mean *lilly white*. And so people who would never be openly racist and nasty to a black person have these lurking notions deep down that somehow black people are different from white people, sexually."

In 1992, I traveled through central Africa with Dr. Harvey Bialy, a molecular biologist and the founding scientific editor of the journal *Bio Technology* who worked as a tropical disease expert in Africa for many years, and Joan Shenton, a British documentary filmmaker researching a documentary on AIDS in Africa for *Dispatches* (Channel Four U.K.), a program that has consistently challenged orthodox views on AIDS. I went because I wanted to see it all with my own eyes, to see how the real picture matched up with the picture I had been given.

That people die of degenerative diseases at an alarming rate in central Africa was not in question. We saw many sick, dying, and dead people during the trip, but the task of trying to decipher just what they were truly dying of struck me as impossible. Often, their doctors didn't even know. In many cases, it seemed not to matter. Death is death, and in Africa, death is common. But AIDS carries with it the same multiple curses of discrimination, terror, guilt, and despondency in Africa that it does in the U.S. And yet in Africa, AIDS diagnoses are given liberally, hastily, with little or no testing to back them up.

Although it was claimed that AIDS originated in Africa, it was not observed at all there until 1983—two years after it had erupted in the United States. By the mid '80s, the "epidemic" was declared. Suddenly, the media was pouring out reports of a continent on the brink of virtual extinction. If the epidemiological projections about AIDS in the U.S. and Europe in the mid '80s were alarming, the ones for Africa were positively hysterical. There was no question: AIDS was bulldozing Africa, taking out entire villages—men, women, and children, changing the demographics of central Africa forever.

Our picture of AIDS in Africa was in large part fueled by the idea that AIDS, or HIV at least, originated there. This theory was based on a few reports that a virus similar to HIV had been found in African blood samples dating as far back as the 1950s. A virus said to be "closely related to" HIV was isolated in the African Green Monkey and before long, the theory evolved that HIV had somehow crossed species, jumping from monkeys to humans through some unidentified mode of transmission. It is difficult to prove where HIV "came from," but it seems no more likely that it came from Africa than anywhere else. As for the stored blood samples, HIV was also found in a Western blood sample dating back to the 1950s. Several leading scholars and researchers have disputed the claims that AIDS originated in Africa and is "decimating" the population.

During our three weeks in Africa we visited Cote d'Ivoire, Uganda, and Kenya, three of the nations said to be the hardest hit by AIDS. As if we were hunting some elusive beast, we tried to follow the footprints, but sometimes they vanished. We got glimpses of insight, pieces of truth that didn't always fit together. In Uganda, a first-rate dictatorship, we had to tread lightly, and seek permission and clearance from various government ministries at every turn. We had been told to pretend we weren't really asking the questions we were asking: Is there really an AIDS epidemic here? What exactly is "AIDS" in Africa? Is it new? Is it the same thing as AIDS in the U.S. and Europe? If it is the same disease caused by the same virus, then why does it manifest itself so differently?

It appears that infectious, often deadly diseases are indeed rising to epidemic levels in Africa, but the lines between the old diseases and the "new" disease, *slim*, are almost hopelessly blurred. Many believe that the statistics have been inflated because AIDS generates far more money in the third world from Western organizations than any other infectious disease. This was clear to us when we were there: Where there was "AIDS" there was money—a brand new clinic, a new Mercedes parked outside, modern testing facilities, high-paying jobs, international conferences. A leading African physician practicing in London, who refused to be named, warned us not to get our hopes up about this trip. "You have no idea what you have taken on," he said on the eve of our departure. "You will never get these doctors to tell you the truth. When they get sent to these AIDS conferences around the world, the per diem they receive is equal to what they earn in a whole year at home."

"AIDS is a perception," said Dr. Kassi Manlan, director general of Health and Social Services in Cote d'Ivoire. "The more you look for it, the more you see it."

CLINIC OF INFECTIOUS DISEASES, TREICHVILLE HOSPITAL, ABIDJAN, COTE D IVOIRE

We asked if we could please see the AIDS wards. The doctor, Aka Kakou, removed his glasses. "You want to see the wards?" he repeated. "Yes," we said. "Could we walk through them, just once?" The doctor rose, and motioned us to follow him. We walked down several long corridors; entire families sat waiting in clusters on straw mats. They looked as if they'd been waiting forever. We entered a room with four cots, all occupied, and stopped at one of them. An old woman sat quietly by the bedside. The doctor shook the patient's foot gently, smiled, and said something. The patient, a young girl, emaciated and wheezing, smiled back. He flipped up the chart hanging on the bedpost, and recited the facts. "Twenty-five years old, HIV-positive, chronic diarrhea, fever, mycosis." He pointed to her toenails, which looked as if they had been badly burned. "Nails atrophied. Not responding to medication...Viola. Le *SIDA*."

We moved on to the next cot, where a young man, equally emaciated, lay on his side. His eyes were wide open and he stared at us intently. The doctor flipped his chart open, "This one has TB. We just got his HIV test back and he is positive, but he doesn't know yet."

"Doesn't know what?"

"That he has AIDS."

We continued down the ward, in and out of rooms, where people lay, often wheezing, or lifeless, wrapped in colorful cloth. Some were HIV-negative, some were positive. They had TB, malaria, meningitis. They had wasting syndrome, diarrhea, fevers, and vomiting. If they were HIV-positive, they were told they had AIDS. If not, then they had whatever they had.

"Is it correct to say," I asked, "that a person has AIDS if they have any one of these old classical diseases, in the presence of HIV?"

"Yes, usually," the doctor said.

"Usually? Do you ever see patients in here who have what you would call AIDS, but test negative for HIV?"

"Negative?" He thinks for a moment and then nods. "Yes, I see some like this."

"How many would you say?"

"Not very many. A few. A few per month, maybe."

RAKAI DISTRICT, UGANDA

We were the only car on the road. Joan and I, seated in the back, stared out the car windows, silenced by the sight. It was as if the whole place had been shredded—a chaos of dust and debris, rotting wood shacks, garbage, people in rags, children in rags. The poverty in Uganda was crushing, total, and unrelenting. As we drove deeper and deeper into the Rakai District, the "AIDS epicenter of the world," all the talk of HIV and T-cells and safer sex started to seem a little absurd. We got out of the car and surveyed what looked like a swamp, with a pipe emerging from it. This was, it turned out, the surrounding villages' water supply. It was also where the sewage was deposited. People looked listless, malnourished. Many of the children had swollen bellies, the telltale sign of malnutrition.

"Don't ask them what they eat," advised one doctor we spoke to, "ask them how often they eat."

The nearest hospital was miles away. There were no cars; the only means of transportation were donkeys and the occasional bicycle. The Ugandan government sets and enforces fees for medication, which most people can't afford. It became clear to us that most people living in the Rakai district had no access to health care whatsoever. Malnutrition, filthy water, diseases left untreated—and the WHO, we learned, had come in with "AIDS educational programs," instructing people how to use condoms?

Scientist Charles E. Gilks, working at the Kenya Medical Research Institute in Nairobi, cautioned in a paper in the *British Medical Journal* in 1991 that the clinical case definition for AIDS in Africa is virtually useless, as it fails to distinguish between infections resulting from HIV, and those such as TB, malaria, and parasitic infections that are endemic in these parts of Africa and that, independent of HIV, themselves lead to severe immune suppression. The results, Gilks warned, is that "substantial numbers of people who are reported as having AIDS may in fact not have AIDS."

One of the diseases that is the most difficult to distinguish from African AIDS is pulmonary tuberculosis, which shares virtually all its symptoms even if HIV is not present.

"The symptoms are the same by and large," said Dr. Okot Nwang, a TB specialist working at Old Mulago Hospital in Kampala, Uganda. "Prolonged fever? The same. Loss of weight, the same. Blood count? A little confusing, CD4 count, both low. So what's the difference? Maybe diarrhea."

From 1985 to 1989, the number of TB patients at Mulago Hospital practically doubled. Most of these were cases of pulmonary TB. In 1993, it was estimated that there were 4 to 5 million cases of highly infectious TB per year worldwide. Annually, 3 million people then died of the disease. According to a study by Nwang, pulmonary TB was most common in the age group of fifteen- to forty-four- year-olds, who comprise 70 to 80 percent of all cases. In light of this, it seems odd that so many doctors make the point that AIDS in Africa is "new" because it is a disease that is killing young people. TB is also killing young people. The ratio of male to female cases with TB is also similar to that of *slim*, two males to one female. How much of what is called AIDS in Africa is TB?

Cote d'Ivoire is a rather prosperous country on the west coast of Africa. From 1984 to 1992, there had been 10,600 declared cases of AIDS there. The capital, Abidjan, a popular tourist resort, is also known as a prostitution and hard drug center of West Africa. In 1992 it was estimated that 50 percent of Abidjan's prostitutes were HIV-positive, and 1.3 million, or 10 percent, of the general population were positive. I was told that in Cote d'Ivoire, AIDS is the leading cause of death among men and the second leading cause among women, the first being maternal mortality.

But the definition of AIDS was problematic and confusing even to African doctors who worked closely with it.

"There is something new, definitely," said Dr. Benoit Soro, an African doctor who carried out research with Dr. Kevin DeCock from the U.S. Centers for Disease Control and Prevention , urging reappraisal of the African AIDS case definition. "Today young people are dying. That was not really the case before, not on this scale. People from all walks of life are dying now—lawyers, doctors. It is not only the poor people in the villages. I think it is dangerous to compare AIDS with the old diseases because AIDS is something new."

Dr. Aka Kakou, an infectious disease specialist working at Treichville Hospital, Abidian, agreed, "None of those diseases are new, it's true, but they are being expressed in a new way, Kakou said. "Diseases that used to be treatable, such as TB, malaria, meningitis, are killing people now. For example, the death rate of meningitis has gone up rather dramatically. We now lose 60 percent of meningitis patients whereas we used to lose only 45 percent. And cerebral malaria is another disease that used to be very rare and is now becoming common. I think that HIV is the underlying cause, of all this. It is exacerbating all these old problems, and rendering them untreatable."

The problem with that theory, however, is that HIV is not a constant factor. A study published in the *British Medical Journal* in 1991, titled "AIDS Surveillance in Africa: A Reappraisal of Case Definitions," studied 1,715 patients admitted to three of Abidjan's main hospitals over a period of three years. All were tested for HIV. Of those, 684 were positive and 1,031 were negative. Of those that were positive, 35 percent fulfilled the WHO definition for AIDS. Of the HIV-negatives, 10 percent met the definition. The point is, many people who have what appears to be *slim* do not have HIV, and *slim* is characterized by general failure to respond to medication or to recover from common sicknesses. Hence there must be exacerbating factors other than HIV.

"This is hairsplitting," said one doctor working at a major hospital in Kampala, Uganda. "There is something new. I don't care if it's HIV or something else but it's something that wasn't there before. I treat people for what symptoms they have when they come to me. That's all that matters."

Most health officials and doctors we interviewed seemed certain that AIDS in Africa is a reality and that it is "something new," but others were less certain. Dr. George Oguna, an infectious disease specialist working in Nairobi, Kenya, when we asked if there is a difference between TB and AIDS, shook his head. "It's all the same," he said. "I've not seen an epidemic of AIDS."

I climbed the dark stairwell of Radio Uganda, a huge complex in central Kampala, and, finally, found Samuel Mulondo's office. Mulondo is one of Uganda's best-known journalists, and his specialty is AIDS. He is a closet dissident: He has doubts about HIV being the real cause of AIDS, and he is exasperated by the hype surrounding AIDS in Africa. But his broadcasts were strictly regulated, and he had to he very careful not to upset the Ugandan authorities.

A few shards of glass clung to the window frame next to his desk. All the windows of the building were similarly shattered, or filled with bullet holes from the civil war.

"I have to slip things in very subtly," he said. "My listeners know how to read between the lines of what I am saying."

Mulondo pointed out that Uganda had been subject to two decades of turmoil, war, decay, and the unparalleled dictatorship and wreckage of General Idi Amin, who was ousted from power in the late 1970s. Uganda had a rather impressive health-care system through the '60s, but it collapsed in the '70s and '80s. Many qualified doctors fled the country leaving it in a state of total disarray, with a terrible shortage of medical supplies.

"People are dying here because they can't afford any basic health care," he said. The poverty is very bad, people are malnourished. I wouldn't connect these deaths to sex, not here. I know a lot of people who are promiscuous and they are not sick.

"Every infection is now called *slim*," he continued angrily, "and it's totally neglected in the rural setting. The stigmatization leads to people not getting medical attention if they are said to have AIDS. Even in the hospitals. It is considered so hopeless that they don't bother to treat them."

Mulondo also did not agree with the statement that middle and upper-class Africans are succumbing at the same rate as poor people in the villages. Mulondo said he had been trying for months to obtain the real figures of AIDS in Uganda but that he couldn't get clearance from the AIDS Information Center, the central bureaucracy that controls the dissemination of statistical information. He requested statistics on the number of HIV infections, number of AIDS cases, number of deaths, and comparative death statistics (meaning how many people died in these regions before AIDS emerged, versus how many after). He received no statistics. "They say they can't give you anything unless it's cleared from the top, at government level," he said. "And they know I'm skeptical of it all so I can't get it. They only tell you what they want you to know."

I also tried to obtain these statistics. Finally, I was told they did not exist. Even in the relatively prosperous Cote d'Ivoire, no actual death statistics are kept.

As in many situations like this, money was also being trapped at an administrative level, and hardly trickling down to the people who needed it. It may well be that—just as it was argued in the West—figures had to be inflated or else nobody would care, but in Africa the consequence of this tactic is far from innocuous.

It has caused a deep psychological wound that one relief worker, Philippe Krynen, calls "AIDS brain," in which people are so convinced they will die they actually get sick, so strong is the belief that a deadly virus has spread like wildfire, and that there is no escaping it.

When Krynen, a French nurse working with AIDS orphans in Kagera, a region of Tanzania near the Uganda border, first came to the area, he told me he realized that the first thing he had to do was get a real answer to the question of how many people were "infected" with HIV. "When I came here," he said, "people had completely given up. Nobody was interested in safe-sex—that's only an option if you think you have a chance. So we decided to test everybody to find out who was not infected. I figured that those who were not infected could become leaders and inspire the others. We tested 150 Tanzanians. We were expecting to find up to 50 percent HIV-positive. We found 5 percent."

But Krynen reasoned that the sample was not representative of the general population, that the age groups and levels of education were different. So he did another round of testing, this time of 842 people—the entire adult population of a village. Of those, 116 were positive, or 13.5 percent. "We had people who were symptomatically AIDS patients," Krynen said. "They were dying of AIDS, but when they were tested and found out they were negative they suddenly rebounded and are now perfectly healthy." Krynen even came across an HIV-positive six-year-old, whose parents are both negative and who has never been to a hospital or received a transfusion. The only time she ever had an injection was as part of UNICEF's basic vaccine program.

"Everybody talks about development in Africa, but there is no such thing," Krynen said. "There is only survival. And now survival is made more difficult because there is no hope for tomorrow.

In the villages where I work, people are totally overwhelmed by the media campaign, which always repeats the same thing—that you're dead. That everybody is infected. This is what they call awareness. We are paying a very high price for this gross exaggeration. The whole community is washed up, despondent, because of this psychological pressure."

Krynen also did a rough count of how many orphans there were in Kagera due to AIDS. In many places in Africa, a child is considered an orphan if not just both parents die, but if one parent dies. Krynen surveyed 160 villages and arrived at a very rough estimate. "Nobody keeps track of the death toll here," he said. "Maybe in some hospitals they do, but they'll only keep the figures for two or three months and then they'll scrap them because they need the paper." He estimated that there would be some 17,500 AIDS orphans in Kagera. "These figures were virtually meaningless," he said. "I made them up myself, but they wound up getting sent off to Kalizizo, and from there to Dar es Salaam, and then to the National AIDS Control Program. Then, to my amazement, they were published as official figures in the WHO 1990 book on African AIDS. After that, every six months the figure just kept jumping up. By now, the figure has more than doubled, based on I don't know what evidence, since these people have never been here. Today they say that there are 50,000 AIDS orphans in Kagera."

Samuel Mulondo agrees: "This safe-sex business is not working. The rate of promiscuity is increasing because people don't give a damn. They've been told that 80 percent are infected, that they're going to die, there's no way out, so people are trying to enjoy themselves. Many people have said to me, 'What's the point? We're all gone anyway. We're dead.' This is the result of these exaggerated AIDS scare campaigns."

"If people die of malaria, it is called AIDS," Krynen said. "If they die of herpes, it is called AIDS. I've even seen people die in accidents and it's been attributed to AIDS. The AIDS figures out of Africa are pure lies, pure estimate."

UGANDA

Gerald wanted me to meet his family. He grabbed my arm and brought me over to their hut. It was dark and musty inside. A young woman carrying a small child emerged. "This is my wife and my daughter," he said. He told us he was an electrician and his monthly salary was about 1,500 Ugandan shillings, or two American dollars. I asked him, and all the others standing around, whether they had seen a new epidemic. Were they clear about what AIDS was? Were they getting any help? Any medical attention? One man laughed. "They come here in those vans every week. They give us condoms for AIDS." Gerald clutched my arm. "Madam," he said, "we are dying because we have no medication."

He walked me over to a nearby hut where his sister, a young woman in her twenties, lay in the dark, alone. She barely stirred when Gerald pulled the cloth off her to reveal an emaciated body and legs covered with sores. I started to ask what she had, but then I realized how futile the question was. Who the hell knows? Certainly no doctor had ever set foot in here. Whatever she "had," it hardly mattered, because there was no money to get her any treatment or medicine at all.

Joan and I pulled out what cash we had and gave it to Gerald, asking that he use it to buy medicine for the girl. We then left the village and drove up a hill, where there was supposedly a clinic. Sam and our driver waited outside as Joan and I pushed open the door and walked in.

The place looked thoroughly abandoned—dark, dirty, a few cots, a few cholera posters, a scale. Surely, we asked, this place isn't in service. We were assured that it was. Suddenly, a woman appeared. "Can I help you?" she asked. She told us she was in charge of the clinic. When we asked her if there were any medical supplies she unlocked a padlocked cabinet which contained a few shelves of various antibiotics.

When Joan returned to Uganda a month later to make her film, she went back to the village and to the clinic on the hill. That was when she learned that the reason the medicine cabinet had been locked was that the government had started to charge money for the medication. She said Gerald had bought medicine for his sister, and that the sores on her legs had almost cleared up and she was walking again.

It was a muggy, rainy day in Rakai, and the car we were driving felt as if it had no tires. The road was a deep red color and stretched out endlessly in front of us as we rattled toward our destination, the Rakai district of Uganda, said to be the AIDS epicenter of the world. In the car with me were two men who work for an organization for AIDS orphans in Rakai and Samuel Mulondo, the Radio Uganda journalist who I had brought with me from Kampala as an interpreter. Sam had taken great care in selecting our driver, explaining that all of the drivers hired through the tourist hotels in Kampala were government informers. "All of them?" I asked, skeptically. "Yes, all of them," he replied.

When Sam and I were planning this excursion in Kampala, a few days earlier, he detailed for me the web of bureaucratic obstacles we would have to navigate before setting off—in order to visit the Rakai district we would need to obtain written permission from the Ministry of Health for the Rakai district, then the Ministry of AIDS, the Ministry of Information, and so on. We spent nearly a whole day crisscrossing Kampala to these various ministries, which all directed us back to one of the others. We needed a written request, a letter from this and that minister granting permission, then a stamp from one of the other ministries, before the next ministry would even look at it. By the end of the day, still not recognizably closer to having obtained permission, we realized we were being kept in a holding pattern. "Okay, let's just go," Sam finally said.

As we left Radio Uganda, Sam caught sight of one of the ministers whose permission we needed. He waved to him across the street, and we quickened our pace to catch up. "I know him," Sam whispered. "Just play dumb Western reporter here to do an AIDS story. Tell him you want to write about the orphans. Nothing else." Sam warned me that a Japanese film crew had been chucked out of the Rakai district and their film confiscated because the government didn't like what they were reporting.

We caught up with the minister and he took us into a large, stone building, up a swirling staircase and into his office, where we sat down in two huge, red leather chairs. He leaned back in his chair and looked at me suspiciously. What did I want? I smiled and said I wanted to write about the orphans, for a young people's magazine in America.

"Young people in particular," I told him, "need to understand how serious the AIDS situation is here. So that perhaps we can prevent the same thing from happening to us."

I couldn't imagine that he would buy that, but he finally grunted and said we could use his name at the next ministry and say he'd given us clearance. We thanked him profusely and hurried out.

Sam sat stonefaced, staring out the car window. The two men from the orphan organization had decided which orphanage to take us to and were instructing the driver. We turned off the main road and started driving through thick, lush terrain on small dirt roads. Finally, we entered a clearing, with a gray stone house built squarely in the middle. A group of about thirty children stood in front of the house, staring fixedly at the car as we approached. When we got out of the car, all the children scurried into neat rows, hands at their sides. The two men introduced us, and the children called out a greeting in unison. When the men gave the word, they dispersed.

I became transfixed by them. They did not seem at all miserable—quite the opposite, they were exuberant, laughing and playing, the bigger ones carrying the smaller ones around on their backs. A few of them came up to me and curtsied, and when I smiled at them, their faces lit up. And there they were, living in an empty house in the bush with nothing, not even parents. The house turned out to be a single room. "Do they all live here?" I asked. Yes. "And where do they sleep?"

"On the floor."

I was ushered inside. Sitting on a bench was an old woman wringing her hands, her eyes fixed on the floor. One of the men explained that six of her ten children had died of AIDS. I sat down to talk to her, and Sam interpreted.

All of them were sons, she said, two of them left no children. The cause of death in all six cases was diarrhea. I asked whether she had ever seen anything like this disease before. She said: "We have been suffering from this illness, diarrhea, for a very long time, but these days it doesn't stop. One of them was so wasted away you couldn't recognize that he was a human being."

"Did they all have HIV?" I asked.

"Yes, apart from one who was thirteen years old. He had malaria. And another one, also age thirteen, who died of typhoid."

She was wearing a bright purple gown. She barely looked at me, her eyes stayed on the floor.

It happened over and over, particularly in these villages, that I was told of a string of AIDS deaths, which were suddenly called malaria, typhoid, TB, or whatever. I had to ask her why, if at least two of her sons died of other diseases, she felt that all six had died of AIDS, but she looked at me blankly and Sam whispered, "She will tell you what she has been told, that it is HIV, and that it is sexually transmitted."

I asked her what the difference was, as far as she could observe, between this AIDS epidemic and diseases people got before. She said, "The difference is that when people got these diseases before, they would get an injection and they would get better. Now they only get worse and they die." I asked about the two sons who had malaria and typhoid. Had they received treatment?

"Yes," she said, "they did. But they died anyway."

It was a story I heard many, many versions of—it seemed clear that, despite medical intervention, people in Uganda were dying young but of several old, familiar diseases, whether they were HIV-positive or not.

In Africa, the danger of misdiagnosed AIDS cases was not the same as in the U.S., namely the threat of highly toxic antiretroviral therapy, such as AZT, but more of a social one. People said to have AIDS were horribly stigmatized, sometimes banished from their villages and left to die, often not treated at all if they did make it to a hospital. This is in addition to the unspeakable terror, and the fixed death sentence that accompanies an AIDS diagnosis. Added to that, there is the guilt associated with the notion that

AIDS, as opposed to other tropical diseases, is a sexually transmitted disease. Blame falls squarely upon the AIDS patient, while the socioeconomic setting is ignored—a scenario that is unsettlingly convenient for the establishment. The appalling conditions of life in Africa are discounted as a health factor and momentum is given to the politically correct, simplistic, and unproven party line that AIDS is going to get everyone, and that sex is the primary cause.

Eighty percent of AIDS is said to be sexually transmitted in Africa. And yet, although 50 percent of the prostitutes in Abidjan, Cote d'Ivoire, for instance, are reported to be infected with HIV, very few have developed AIDS. At the major infectious disease clinic in Abidjan, which handles most of Abidjan's AIDS cases, the director told us that he hardly saw any cases of AIDS in prostitutes. Nor did he see any IV-drug users or gay men. Likewise in Kenya, where 80 percent of the prostitutes were said to be infected with HIV, very few have AIDS. A lab technician we spoke to in Nairobi, Kenya, who worked with HIV testing, confirmed, "Most people with HIV here in Africa stay healthy. The prostitutes have remained healthy."

One doctor in Nairobi, who treats many AIDS patients, Dr. Manohar Nene, was quite upset about the emphasis on sex as opposed to other factors. "We have psychologically upset the sexually active population of the world. If you upset people's notion of sex, it is terribly disruptive."

Nene said he does not believe AIDS, or HIV at least, is sexually transmitted, because the number of infected cells in semen is so low.

Also, he said. "When you make people feel guilty about sex, which is a natural thing, you add a stress, and stress can cause disease." A poster in the lobby we passed on the way to his office showed a heart with a worm crawling through it. It read, "Careless sex is a fruit with a worm in it. AIDS."

We left and started to walk toward the car and one of the two men said, "Somebody in the next village has just died of slim. We want to take you there."

I looked at Sam, whose face betrayed nothing.

"Somebody just died?"

"Yes," he said. "Let's go."

I hesitated before getting in the car. Why were they so eager for me to see a corpse?

We drove deeper into the bush until we reached another clearing.

It contained a little village, with a small cluster of huts. There was garbage everywhere, and plastic bowls in bright colors, and coils of black smoke rising here and there, but no food. It was very quiet; the only sound was the tap of the rain. We walked up to one of the huts. Inside, the floor of the hut was filled with women sitting on the floor. In the middle of the hut, against the wall, was a coffin. A candle and a picture of Christ hung over it. One older woman was draped over the coffin, sobbing, the others sat very still and quiet, looking on. Outside, another twenty women gathered.

I felt very uncomfortable and I whispered to one of the men, "Thank you, but can we go now?" But he started motioning me into the hut, pointing to the coffin. He virtually pushed me up to the doorway where I stood transfixed as one of the women slowly lifted the lid of the coffin and then started to peel away the layers of white cloth that covered the dead man's face. When the crying woman caught sight of her son's face, she let out a loud cry and one of the other women gripped her. His face was gaunt and his nostrils were stuffed with cotton. He looked about thirty.

I don't know anything about the man, his history, or the cause of his death. I don't know whether he died of AIDS. But it struck me as slightly odd that the two gentlemen from the AIDS organization seemed so intent on showing me this dead man, and they kept saying, over and over, that he had died of AIDS. I don't know whether he had even been to a hospital, had ever been tested for HIV. But they did say that he hadn't been sick for long, which was rather typical. Scores of men getting sick and dying within a matter of months is not a description that fits what we in the West refer to as AIDS. Are there other diseases that behave radically differently on different continents?

"No," noted Bialy later. "Why should African AIDS be any different than AIDS in any other country? Do we have French AIDS? Brazilian AIDS? The definition of this thing gets more and more nebulous all the time. At this point, you may as well call anything AIDS."

KAMPALA, UGANDA

There was an herbal doctor who treated AIDS patients in Kampala whom Sam wanted me to meet. Downtown Kampala is dusty, torn, and chaotic, as if recently bombed. I followed Sam through the streets and down an alleyway, over which hung a crooked sign that read "Clinic for AIDS Research." Like everything in Uganda, the doctor's office was cramped, dark, and rickety. People were packed into the tiny area like commuters at rush hour. We had to push our way through to the doctor, who sat in a little fluorescent-lit cubicle.

Sam introduced me, and the doctor shook my hand and started talking about his treatments. He had learned the recipes from his grandfather, and he claimed to be the only doctor in Kampala who was having success with AIDS patients. He knew how to stop the diarrhea. He hollered to an assistant and a hand holding a bottle of medicine came through a side window covered by a little red curtain. He held up the bottle. "This is for diarrhea," he said. It was a mixture of honey and herbs. Then he started hollering

Serious Adverse Events
An Uncensored History of AIDS

again, and more and more bottles came through the window, until he was surrounded by bottles. They had funny names on the labels such as "Red Hot Devil Liquid."

He said he treated several hundred patients per day. People were clamoring toward the back room, where the bottles were kept in huge baskets. One man grabbed my arm and wouldn't let me go until he had convinced me that the doctor had cured him and several of his friends of *slim*.

One can only hope. Meanwhile, I noted that AZT was virtually nonexistent in Africa. I didn't meet a single doctor who was even remotely interested in AZT. As one doctor put it, "it doesn't work, does it? So it's just as well that we can't afford it."

"AZT does not cure AIDS, is very expensive, and causes too many complications," said Dr. Kassi Manlan, director general of health and social services for Cote d'Ivoire, explaining why Cote d'Ivoire does not use AZT for AIDS. The entire annual health-care budget for the country would be spent if just 1,000 people were treated with AZT.

ENTEBBE, KAMPALA

It was an eerie drive from the airport in Entebbe back to the hotel in Kampala. Prior to Idi Amin, prior to the last three decades, Uganda was known as "The Pearl of Africa," and was said to be one of the most beautiful places on earth. Some say that the Garden of Eden was in Uganda. Now it is one of the poorest, most disease-ridden countries in Africa. The road to Kampala was lined with people building and selling coffins. Simple wooden boxes with black crosses on the front.

Sam and I were looking for a place to have lunch in downtown Kampala. We went to a roadside cafe and ordered grilled chicken.

Upon asking for a toilet, I was shown through the kitchen and into the backyard, where a whole separate world was bubbling. There were chicken parts everywhere—heads, feet, feathers, and live chickens pecking in the mud—women standing over vats of dirty water, rinsing potatoes in them, coils of black smoke, and a rancid, oily-stench. The toilet was a shack with a hole in the ground. In fact, every toilet I saw in Uganda, except in the hotel, was a hole in the ground. I went to inspect the toilets at Mulago hospital, the major hospital in Kampala, and even there—a hole in the floor, covered in excrement and buzzing with flies.

Although the poverty in Uganda was shocking and brutal, it wasn't the most distressing thing about it. The most distressing thing was the lack of any kind of infrastructure. It seemed like chaos on earth, genuine chaos. When Joan and I were sitting in the airport, waiting to fly to Nairobi, I looked up and noticed the airport lounge had no ceiling. All the wiring was hanging down, plaster falling. It seemed to be symbolic of all of Uganda. The government had crushed the country, the people, and then vanished and left a population steeped in lawlessness, chaos, and poverty. Each time we hired a driver to go on an excursion, they were manic about getting on the road back to Kampala by mid-afternoon—so as not to be driving after dark. They feared being robbed, even killed on the road. Nobody would drive after dark. "You'd have to be crazy," said one driver.

The bank in our hotel was robbed one morning, just as I was walking toward it. There were power failures constantly. No medical supplies, even in the hospitals. People were crammed throughout the corridors of the hospitals, waiting, maybe for days, to get any attention, and even then, what attention? What medication they had was poor quality, often too strong, unspecific, and ineffective. People bought prescription medications from little shacks called drugstores that had smuggled them from God knows where. Deaths were not counted, except maybe at some hospitals, but many people just died in the villages. It was not known how many people had died in any given year, much less what the cause of death had been. To try to make sense out of AIDS, with HIV tests and T-cell counts and clinical case definitions, in this chaos seemed hopeless; and to saddle them with this unproven, unwarranted death sentence and terror seemed almost cruel. The first thing we heard upon arriving in Mombasa, Kenya, was from Joan's friend who picked us up at the train station. "Terrible," he said, shaking his head. "I just heard on the radio that a young woman jumped to her death from a hospital roof because she got the results of her test and she was HIV-positive."

Seated next to us on the plane from Kenya back to London was a British gentleman who had been working with a water restoration program in Kenya for six months.

"That must have been interesting," I said. "Is the water really bad in Kenya?"

"Oh, my God," he said. "You should have seen it when we got there. People were so sick."

"Sick?" we said.

"Mmm. They had the most atrocious diarrhea and vomiting and abdominal pains."

I stared at him.

"How long had this been going on," I asked.

"Oh, about ten years."

"And did the symptoms subside when you cleaned the water?"

"Oh, absolutely."

Joan and I looked at each other, sighed and ordered a drink. Beneath us, Africa was disappearing.

The first time I interviewed Kary Mullis was in 1991, in the bar of a hotel somewhere in New Jersey while a blizzard raged outside. His demeanor surprised me. Here was a man responsible for one of the greatest scientific inventions of the century—the mass duplication of DNA—and he swaggered in wearing jeans, cracking jokes in a sharp Southern accent, ordering drinks, and utterly lacking that sterile, statesmanlike aura that usually looms over men of science.

Instead, Mullis, who has been described in the press as possessing a "creative nonconformity that verges on the lunatic," struck me as a person with a pure and insatiable curiosity. He had as many questions for me as I had for him. For instance, at the end of the interview, he asked me to articulate why it would matter if I were to discover that the hotel lobby, the bar, the bartender, the drinks, and our conversation had all been an electronic mirage.

Mullis's invention of polymerase chain reaction (PCR) won him the Nobel Prize in chemistry in 1993. PCR is a remarkably simple yet revolutionary method of selectively multiplying and mass-producing specific DNA segments in just hours. Previously, DNA could be multiplied, but not isolated, and the development of an isolation technique was a radical breakthrough. Scientists can now undertake everything from detecting hereditary cancers in fetuses, to solving impossible murder mysteries, to retracing the very depths of evolution. The London *Observer* trumpeted: "Not since James Watt walked across Glasgow Green in 1765 and realized that the secondary steam condenser would transform steam power, an inspiration that set loose the industrial revolution, has a single, momentous idea been so well recorded in time and place."

Now there could be precise biological vision where there used to be darkness. The PCR machine is now a staple of every biology laboratory allowing speculation to crystallize into fact. An American soldier killed in Vietnam, for instance, was identified after more than a generation by matching the DNA in a lock of his baby hair to a single bone found on the battlefield. A man who had served nine years in prison for a rape and murder he did not commit was released thanks to a PCR test on a dried speck of semen taken from the crime scene. President Lincoln's suspected genetic disease, Marfan's syndrome, can finally be diagnosed based on his stored bone fragments. The FBI knew quickly that PCR would make it possible to identify extortionists by the DNA from their salvia left on the flap of an envelope, and even ancient DNA from dinosaurs can be resurrected and studied. In fact, PCR was the conceptual root of Michael Crichton's blockbuster novel *Jurassic Park*.

And of course, PCR has also had a great impact on HIV research. PCR can, among other things, detect HIV in people who test negative to the HIV antibody test.

The word "eccentric" seems to come up often in connection with Mullis name: His first published scientific paper, in the premier scientific journal *Nature* in 1986, described how he viewed the universe while on LSD—packed with black holes containing antimatter, for which time runs backward. He has been known to show photographs of nude girlfriends during his lectures, their bodies traced with Mandelbrot fractal patterns. And as a side project, he developed a company that sells lockets containing the DNA of rock stars. But it was his views on AIDS that really set the scientific establishment fuming.

Mullis, like Peter Duesberg, does not believe that AIDS is caused by the retrovirus HIV. He is long-standing member of the Group for the Reappraisal of the HIV-AIDS Hypothesis, the 2,300-member protest organization pushing for a re-examination of the cause of AIDS.

One of Duesberg's strongest arguments in the debate has been that the HIV virus is barely detectable in people who suffer from AIDS. Ironically, when PCR was applied to HIV research, around 1989, researchers claimed to have put this complaint to rest. Using the new technology, they were suddenly able to see viral particles in the quantities they couldn't see before. Scientific articles poured forth stating that HIV was now 100 times more prevalent than was previously thought. But Mullis himself was unimpressed. "PCR made it easier to see that certain people are infected with HIV," he noted in 1992, "and some of those people came down with symptoms of AIDS. But that doesn't begin even to answer the question, 'Does HIV cause it?'"

"The mystery of that damn virus," he said, "has been generated by the $2 billion a year they spend on it. You take any other virus, and spend $2 billion, and you can make up some great mysteries about it, too."

"Human beings are full of retroviruses. We don't know if it's hundreds, or thousands, or hundred of thousands. We've only recently started to look for them. But they've never killed anybody before. People have always survived retroviruses."

"We're scientists," noted Mullis the first time I spoke with him. "Scientists don't believe, they have evidence. We don't believe like Christians believe, our souls are not on the line. I've never seen anything like this."

"And yet," he continued, "I think most of them have done it innocently. They're not evil people, they're just trying to do their job. My reading of most virologists is that they are neurotic. They have been co-opted over a long period of time by a system that is very large, very complex. The system that they have been gaining their information from for a long time has been progressively more and more unreliable. What they call fact is what is published in their journals by them, and that is becoming more and more muddled and more neurotic.... I have asked a lot of really intelligent people—I get around these days, and I talk to the very best scientists. I've talked to people at the CDC, the NIH, you name it. I generally say, 'Excuse me, but as an independent scientist I often have to write papers on AIDS for the company I'm hired to work for, and the first sentence I write is often, 'HIV is the causative agent in AIDS.' Now, I would like to be able to reference that.'"

"'Reference?' they ask."

"And I say, 'Yes, you know, a reference. Would you mind writing down for me the references that you think, if I read them, I would agree with that statement. I mean, I don't want it to be my idea.' I have never gotten a straight answer to that question from any virologist. They say 'Yes, yes, of course. As soon as I get back to my office I'll have that for you.' And I call them back, and they don't have it. There is no such body of knowledge. The thing has been contrived from newspaper reports, word of mouth, agreement in the back rooms of the virology labs—whatever they do when all ten thousand of them get together in Europe and have their big HIV meeting. It doesn't derive from anything that could be called scientific tradition. The only goddamn person that ever sent me anything back was a virologist from this company called Diagnostic Products. And do you know what he sent me? He sent me the attack that Robin Weiss made on Duesberg in *Nature*!

All that article said was Peter Duesberg is a fool. We don't need to look at the virus. We don't need to look at the facts, at the spread of AIDS, nothing. I couldn't believe it."

Like so many great scientific discoveries, the ideas for PCR came suddenly, as if by direct transmission from another realm. It was during a late-night drive in 1984, the same year, ironically, that HIV was announced to be the cause of AIDS.

"I was just driving and thinking about ideas and suddenly I saw it," Mullis recalls. "I saw the polymerase chain reaction as clear as if it were up on a blackboard in my head, so I pulled over and started scribbling." A chemist friend of his was asleep in the car, and, as Mullis described in a special edition of *Scientific American*: "Jennifer objected groggily to the delay and the light, but I exclaimed I had discovered something fantastic. Unimpressed, she went back to sleep."

Mullis kept scribbling calculations, right there in the car, until the formula for DNA amplification was complete. The calculation was based on the concept of "reiterative exponential growth processes," which Mullis had picked up from working with computer programs. After much table-pounding, he convinced the small California biotech company he was working for, Cetus, that he was on to something. Good thing they finally listened: They sold the patent for PCR to Hoffman-LaRoche for $300 million—the most money ever paid for a patent. Mullis meanwhile received a $10,000 bonus.

Mullis's mother reports that as a child, her lively son got into all kinds of trouble—shutting down the house's electricity, building rockets, and blasting small frogs hundreds of feet into the air. These days, he likes to surf, Rollerblade, take pictures, party with his friends—most of whom are not scientists—and above all, he loves to write.

Mullis is notoriously difficult to track down and interview. I had left several messages on his answering machine at home, but had gotten no response. Finally, I called him in the late evening and he picked up, in the middle of bidding farewell to some dinner guests. He insisted he would not give me an interview, but after a while, a conversation was underway, and I asked if I couldn't just please turn my tape recorder on. "Oh what the hell," he muttered. "Turn the fucker on."

Our talk focused on AIDS. Though Mullis has not been particularly vocal about his HIV skepticism, his convictions have not been muddled or softened by his recent success and mainstream acceptability. He seems to revel in his newly acquired power. "They can't pooh-pooh me now, because of who I am," he says with a chuckle. And by all accounts, he's using that power effectively.

When ABC's Nightline approached Mullis about participating in a documentary on himself, he instead urged them to focus their attention on the HIV debate. "That's a much more important story," he told the producers, who up to that point had never acknowledged the controversy. In the end, Nightline ran a two-part series, the first on Kary Mullis, the second on the HIV debate. Mullis was hired by ABC for a two-week period, to act as their scientific consultant and direct them to sources.

The show was superb, and represented a historic turning point, the end of a seven-year media blackout on the HIV debate. But it still didn't fulfill Mullis's ultimate fantasy. "What ABC needs to do," said Mullis, "is talk to [Chairman of the National Institutes of Allergy and Infectious Diseases Dr. Anthony] Fauci and Gallo and show that they're assholes, which I could do in ten minutes."

But, I point outed, Gallo would refuse to discuss the HIV debate, just as he's always done.

"I know he will," Mullis shoots back, anger rising in his voice. "But you know what? I would be willing to chase the little bastard from his car to his office and say, 'This is Kary Mullis trying to ask you a goddamn simple question,' and let the cameras follow. If people think I'm a crazy person, that's okay. But here's a Nobel Prize-winner trying to ask a simple question from those who spent $22 billion and killed 100,000 people. It has to be on TV. It's a visual thing. I'm not unwilling to do something like that."

He pauses, then continues. "And I don't care about making an ass of myself, because most people realize I am one."

While many people, even within the ranks of the HIV dissidents, tried to distance themselves from the controversial Peter Duesberg, Mullis defends him passionately and seems genuinely concerned about his fate. "I was trying to stress this point to the ABC people" he says, "that Peter has been abused seriously by the scientific establishment, to the point where he can't even do any research. Not only that, but his whole life is pretty much in disarray because of this, and it is only because he has refused to compromise his scientific moral standards. There ought to be some goddamn private foundation in the country, that would say, 'Well, we'll move in where the NIH dropped off. We'll take care of it. You just keep right on saying what you're saying, Peter. We think you're an asshole, and we think you are wrong, but you're the only dissenter, and we need one, because it's science, it's not religion.'"

"I am waiting to be convinced that we're wrong," Mullis continued. "I know it ain't going to happen. But if it does, I will tell you this much—I will be the first person to admit it. A lot of people studying this disease are looking for the clever little pathways they can piece together, that will show how this works. Like, 'What if this molecule was produced by this one and then this one by this one, and then what if this one and that one induce this one'—that stuff becomes, after two molecules, conjecture of the rankest kind. People who sit there and talk about it don't realize that molecules themselves are somewhat hypothetical, and that their interactions are more so, and that the biological reactions are even more so. You don't need to look that far. You don't discover the cause of something like AIDS by dealing with incredibly obscure things. You just look at what the hell is going on. Well, here's a bunch of people that are practicing a new set of behavioral norms. Apparently it didn't work because a lot of them got sick. That's the conclusion. You don't necessarily know why it happened. But you start there."

Mullis points out that transportation and sheer population growth have greatly increased the number of other human beings a person is likely to come into contact with during the course of a lifetime, and argues that "bathhouse cultures of some metropolitan gay communities" enabled an unprecedented exchange of infectious viruses. Such a viral overload, Mullis suggests, may trigger an immune chain reaction that could destabilize or debilitate immune function. Transfusion of blood from one such highly infected individual, he argues further, could transfer enough viruses to cause immune dysfunction in the recipient. He disagrees with Duesberg's idea that AIDS is a toxicological syndrome, caused by drugs, but says that he feels both of their theories "ought to be tested at least."

He is aware that this view of AIDS—one that encompasses each person's history or "lifestyle"—is rejected by virtually all AIDS organizations, researchers, and activists, who consider it "blaming the victim." "It's not blaming the victim," Mullis argues.

"It's not anybody's fault. They just did something that didn't work, that's all." Commenting on the hostility with which these ideas are met, Mullis says, "People don't want to hear from somebody like me who's not a member of their society. They say to me, 'You don't know shit about this, Mullis.' People say to me, 'How many people have you seen die of this disease?' They say, 'You don't know what causes it because you've never watched them die.'"

I ask Mullis why he ever became involved in this debate, particularly since he's an independent scientist, with no financial or professional stake in either point of view.

"I was driving one night," Mullis explains, "must have been around 1987, from Berkeley down to La Jolla, and I was trying to stay awake. I turned on public radio and there was Peter Duesberg. I knew who he was and I knew there was some controversy about him, but I didn't know any details. And I just listened. And I said this man is pretty damn intelligent."

Mullis invited Duesberg to speak at the chemistry conference he was organizing. "At first the audience was ready to jeer him," Mullis recalls. "The questions at first were kind of like 'you asshole.' By the time the two hours were up, everybody was totally convinced that he had a good case. After the animosity wears off—which takes longer as he becomes more of a martyr—people realize this man knows what the hell's going on and nobody else does. Afterward, everybody came to my house for a party. I've got beautiful pictures of Peter, swimming in the ocean without a wet suit."

Referring to the guardians of the HIV establishment, such as Gallo and Fauci, Mullis suddenly turns from rage to pity. "I feel sorry for 'em," he admits. "I want to have the story unveiled, but you know what? I'm just not the kick-'em-in-the-balls kind of guy. I'm a moral person, but I'm not a crusader. I think it's a terrible tragedy that it's happened. There are some terrible motivations of humans involved in this, and Gallo and Fauci have got to be some of the worst."

"Personally, I want to see those fuckers pay for it a little bit. I want to see them lose their position. I want to see their goddamn children have to go to junior college. I mean, who do we care about? Do we care about these people that are HIV-positive whose lives have been ruined? Those are the people I'm the most concerned about. Every night I think about this. I think, what is my interest in this? Why do I care? I don't know anybody dying of it. They're right about that. Well, except one of my girlfriend's brothers died of it, and I think he died of AZT."

At this point, Mullis voice starts to crack. "The horror of it is every goddamn thing you look at, if you look at it through the glasses that you've developed through looking at this thing, seems pretty scary to me. Look at the oncogene people and I go, oh yeah, I know what they are doing. Same stuff. Oncogenes don't have anything to do with cancer. Radiation probably doesn't have anything to do with stopping cancer. The drugs that we use on people—all those goddamn horrible poisons—they're no less toxic than AZT. And we are doing it to everybody. Everybody's aunt is being radiated once a goddamn month and given drugs that are going to kill her. We're dealing with a bunch of witch doctors. The whole medical profession—except for the people that patch you up when you get a broken leg or you have a plumbing problem—is really fucked. It's just a bunch of people that have become socially important and very rich by thinking about the fact that they might be able to cure the diseases that actually cause people in our society to die. And they can't do shit about it. It's scary, that's what it is."

He takes a deep breath, and I realize that on the other end of the phone, Kary Mullis, Nobel laureate, pioneer of the DNA revolution, has started to cry. "God, I hate this kind of crap. I really don't want to write about it. I'd like to write about something that's easy to write about, where you don't have to come up with a conclusion in the end. I've been writing about my boyhood, when I was a little kid back on my grandfather's farm where we didn't know about black widow spiders or all that stuff. But writing about that is so easy. Sometimes in the morning, when it's a good surf, I go out there, and I don't feel like it's a bad world. I think it's a good world, the sun is shining. I'm really optimistic in the mornings. But, you know, it's not because of you calling me. It's just thinking about this issue, it just drives me to—I'm making tears thinking about it. I don't see how to deal with it. I can't possibly write a book that will describe it to somebody. You can't do a damn 22.8-minute TV thing that is going to have any effect except to get somebody to shoot through my window and hit me. I feel like I'm on a hostile planet."

Once, at a community forum meeting in New York, a leading AIDS activist, when asked about whether Mullis shouldn't be taken seriously, answered that he should not, for he is a "sexist pig." This was based on something Mullis allegedly said upon receiving the Nobel prize—that the prize would be "a great way to pick up babes." I present Mullis with this logic.

"They just want to show that I'm not politically correct," he says. "Well I'm not. And the reason is that I already got my money from the Swedes, right? I'm done, I'm fixed. I'm a free agent, and it is the most wonderful feeling. There is nobody on the planet that can fuck with me. And I can say exactly what I feel about any issue and I'm going to do that. A lot of people are not going to like it, but a lot of people are going to say, 'Well, that's really cool that you said that.' And I'm not really going to care about the people who don't like it."

The story first rippled through every news media outlet in the fall of 1996: Prescription-drug "cocktails" were having such a dramatic impact on AIDS that the very nature of the disease was being reversed. People were springing back from their deathbeds, worried now not about dying but about living—about credit card balances and career prospects and life insurance policies already sold. Having spent all those years preparing to die, some people found the idea of living almost unsettling. One activist dubbed this new journalistic phenomenon "I'm-Gonna-Live-and-I-Have-Nothing-to-Wear." *Newsweek's* cover asked whether this was "The End of AIDS?" *Time* named Dr. David Ho, the virologist who paved the way for the current drug "cocktail" revolution, as the Man of the Year for 1996.

Two articles in particular played major roles in launching this new optimism, because they were written by HIV-positive journalists who were themselves taking the drugs: Andrew Sullivan, former editor of the *New Republic,* wrote a lengthy personal cover essay for the *New York Times Magazine* entitled "When Plagues End—Notes on the Twilight of an Epidemic," and David Sanford of the *Wall Street Journal* penned a front-page article heading "Last Year, This Editor Wrote His Own Obituary."

Sullivan's article was met with great jubilation, as well as fury. Sullivan explored his own experience with AIDS—the deaths he witnessed, the fear he's felt, the onslaught of grief that anybody involved in this epidemic goes trough—but the occasion of the article was the new pharmaceuticals. People were taking an array of different drugs in more than 100 combinations. Sullivan, despite all the qualifiers in his piece, was a believer. "The power of the newest drugs, called protease inhibitors," he wrote, "and the even greater power of those in the pipeline, is such that a diagnosis of HIV infection is not just different in degree today than, say, five years ago. It is different in kind. It no longer signifies death. It merely signifies illness." He went on to write: "I realized that my diagnosis was no different in kind than the diagnosis every mortal being lives with—only different in degree. By larger and larger measures, I began to see the condition not as something constricting, but as something liberating... liberating because an awareness of the inevitability of death is always the surest way to an awareness of the tangibility of life."

Writer and activist Richard Berkowitz described the streets of Greenwich Village on November 10, the day Sullivan's article was published: "I went to a gay cinema, and almost everybody had a copy. Everyone was talking about it. People were calling their mothers, weeping. Seeing those words on the cover of the *New York Times* like that was almost Biblical. The desperation to believe it is so huge."

Science reporter Jon Cohen was skeptical about the new drugs and one of the most prominent voices to assail Sullivan. In the online magazine *Slate*, Cohen insisted that only a vaccine could signal the end of AIDS: "Never in the annals of medicine has a viral plague been stopped by any therapy."

For his part, Sullivan felt his intended message was misconstrued. In an exchange with me, he wrote, "My *Times* piece was a first attempt to conceive of a world after AIDS. It was titled 'When Plagues End,' not 'The Plague Has Ended.' It also talked about the end of a 'plague,' not the end of a disease. 'Plague' I define as something unstoppable, out of our control completely, affecting everyone indiscriminately. That phase clearly has ended, and it raises a host of fascinating and difficult questions."

All the stories about the new drug combinations—including Sullivan's—were laced with caveats: Some people "fail" on the drugs, and many cannot afford them. But the core caveat is so monumental that it undermines the central premise. Time has not borne out whether the Lazarus effect of these new drugs will last. Rebounding from severe illness is one thing, "ending" AIDS is altogether another. Yet Sullivan seemed to believe that the resistance to imagining an end to AIDS is psychological, not scientific in nature. "I do think that Camus' insight that at the end of plagues some people refuse to accept it because they have come to need the experience emotionally is a profound one," he wrote to me. "I know of no other disease where patient activists are so keen to tell people to avoid treatment."

Historically, however, "patient activism" in AIDS was built on a philosophy of "Drugs Into Bodies," meaning that people with HIV did not have time to wait and see whether drugs worked or not, but had to gamble. They did, and in the first round of gambling—with AZT—they undeniably lost. This time around there was no consensus. For all the hype and excitement surrounding the new drugs, skeptical voices were heard early on. Both AIDS organizations and treatment activists protested the hype emanating from the Vancouver AIDS conference in 1996, which centered on Ho's announcement that he had used drug combinations to bring several patients down to "undetectable" levels of HIV, as measured by a so-called "viral load" test. Ho had expressed an "evangelical" zeal, as the *Wall Street Journal*'s put it, to get HIV-positive people on drug combinations as soon as possible.

He speculated that after two or three years of treatment, the virus might be eradicated and patients could go off the drugs.

Meanwhile, the viral-load test replaced the T-cell count as a barometer for illness. But as treatment activist Mike Barr reported in *POZ* magazine early in the cocktail craze, an "undetectable" viral load merely means a number below an *arbitrary* cut-off point of 400 to 500 copies of HIV RNA per milliliter of blood. Some people have reached those levels on other drugs, like AZT and D4T, without getting any healthier. In other words, the viral-load test was problematic and was considered so from the beginning. "I used this HIV viral-load test since it became available," Dr. Donald Abrams, assistant director of the AIDS program at San Francisco General Hospital, said in 1997, "but I'm not convinced that I really, truly understand its correlation with clinical outcome." One Los Angeles company sold viral-load tests for $10 during a trial period to induce sales; at the time the test sold for $200 to $300.

"I've heard every version—people swearing by these drugs and people writhing on the floor in agony," noted the late James Scutero, who founded the once popular *mischealthaids.org* discussion group.

Indeed, AIDS seemed in a state of suspension, for there were striking parallels between the cocktail craze and the emergence of AZT in the late '80s. "I suffer from historical perspective," noted Abrams of San Francisco General, who rarely prescribed the new drugs. "I remember 1987, when AZT first became available. I was not convinced that it was the be-all and end-all. That stance was very unpopular, and then over the course of ten years more and more people started to come around."

Sean Strub, chairman and founder of *POZ*, is living proof that the new therapies work wonders for some. "I probably would be dead if these drugs hadn't come along," he told me over lunch in 1997. "A year and a half ago, I had Kaposi's sarcoma in my lungs and was taking chemotherapy every two weeks. I had lesions all over my face. Then I started combinations and within weeks it turned me around."

But Strub did not believe in 1997 that asymptomatic people should take the new drugs. "I have so many friends who waited—wisely so—with AZT. Those same cautious people are now going on cocktails. I try to stop them, but it's difficult." At the same time, he couldn't help wondering if the parallels with AZT would be played out to a tragic conclusion. "My friends who were diagnosed at the same time I was, and who went on AZT, are virtually all dead today," he said. "Those of us who held out are alive."

It's telling, and perfectly symbolic, that when AIDS researcher David Ho's face appeared on the cover of *Time* as Man of the Year, 1996, you couldn't see his eyes. Instead, a colorful swirl meant to represent HIV filled his glasses. George Orwell used precisely this image—a man whose eyes are gone, whose glasses have been filled with the refracting light of his ideology—to convey the triumph of politics over truth in his famous essay, "Politics and the English Language."

Ho, then the newly appointed director of the Aaron Diamond AIDS Research Center in New York, was suddenly catapulted to a degree of fame that no other AIDS researcher had ever attained, and it gave him an oracular power over the press and the AIDS community. The relentlessly-driven son of Chinese immigrants, he was a man singularly obsessed with HIV, and his vision was to attack it with a ferocity never before imagined—to bomb it with not one drug, or two, but a literal hail. He popularized and largely pioneered the idea that would make such pharmaceutical bombing seem rational: that HIV, far from being the cryptic, latent, quiet virus most researchers thought it was, was in fact "replicating furiously," from the very moment of infection. The immune system, he claimed, fought back valiantly, mass-producing immune system cells in an effort to defend itself, but in the end, the virus would win the battle, and the immune system would collapse.

The only rational attack, therefore, was to begin treatment as early as possible, to defeat the virus. Ho was a man of simple concepts, and the one that would alter history went like this: Hit hard, hit early.

Ho's seductive experiment, news of which spread to newspapers around the world before it was ever completed, was to knock back HIV to the point of being "undetectable," then take the patients off the "cocktail" of drugs, with HIV, hopefully, banished for good. His recipe for a cure, a word that was heavily implied if semantically avoided, was to create a blitzkrieg of chemicals—a mixture of old AIDS drugs like AZT with the new class of drugs waiting in the pipeline called "protease inhibitors"—to annihilate HIV in the bloodstream. Protease inhibitors had been researched since the early '90s by the major drug companies, several of which came close to abandoning the effort because the drugs did not work against HIV. But Ho was convinced that his new approach of mixing several drugs would work where no single drug had succeeded, and that curing AIDS was a simple matter of eradicating HIV.

Magazines and newspapers took Ho's central metaphor and reprinted it without a second thought: AIDS is like a full sink with the drain open; the water pours in from the tap at a slightly slower rate than it drains away. Eventually, the water—the T-cells of the immune system—will drain away enough to cause the immune system collapse known as AIDS.

David Ho, *Time* magazine gushed, "fundamentally changed the way scientists looked at the AIDS virus.... His pioneering experiments with protease inhibitors helped clarify how the virus ultimately overwhelms the immune system.... Mathematical models suggest that patients caught early enough might be virus-free within two or three years."

Ho, *Time* concluded, delivered "what may be the most important fact about AIDS: It is not invincible."

Based largely on a single research paper, protease inhibitors received lightning-quick FDA approval and poured onto the market.

The mass media declared AIDS to be "over," albeit with a question mark floating overhead. A new euphoria filled the air, and David Ho spawned a multibillion-dollar drug industry.

Amidst the excitement, however, something was overlooked. Ho's mathematical model was wrong.

The new drugs, unlike the prior generation, AZT, ddI, and d4T, were very specific in their ability to inhibit HIV's crucial protease—DNA and protein are the basics of life, and protease are what control the proteins, turn them on and off, and process them.

The turning point for the new drugs came in 1995, when Ho and another scientist, Dr. George Shaw, co-authored a paper, published in the eminent scientific journal *Nature*, in which he detailed his new vision of HIV, AIDS, and the immune system. On the day the paper was published, a press conference was held. The "new model" was coupled with the new drugs, and a new technology took center stage—so-called "viral load" testing. Rather than focus on physical symptoms, the new craze was to take the drugs and measure your viral load (the amount of virus in the blood) and CD4 cells, now considered a barometer for the immune system's health. The new drug regimens were supposed to lower the former and raise the latter. The concept was: Beat back the bad guys (HIV-infected cells), and the good guys (CD4 cells) will win.

The central puzzle of HIV research up until that point had been how the HIV virus could cause AIDS, when it infected only a trivial number of T-cells—the cells AIDS patients were deficient in. As one researcher said, it was a crime scene with many more bodies than bullets. But Ho's faith in the destructive ability of HIV was so deep that he produced buttons that he wore and distributed at an AIDS conference in 1995 that said "It's the Virus, Stupid."

Ho is not a mathematician, but nevertheless he contrived a mathematical model, in consultation with mathematicians, on which he would base his entire premise. The model was supposed to demonstrate that HIV killed healthy cells slightly faster than they were able to replenish themselves, but the math was so dubious that very few AIDS researchers could grasp it enough to either validate or reject it. Nobody bothered to try.

Meanwhile, the "breakthrough" provided hope to two main players: HIV-positive people could hope for a new lease on life, and the drug companies could sell drugs like never before. They could even keep their customers convinced, through the AIDS care-network itself, that total compliance with the draconian discipline of the cocktail was the only path to heroic survival. Miss one pill, the new wisdom held, and HIV, enigmatically, will "mutate."

Those who know Ho, or have met him, describe him on the one hand as "a nice guy," and on the other as a man totally bereft of personality. But whatever his personal characteristics, he certainly played a pivotal role in not just AIDS history but medical history. It was at an AIDS science conference in Florida in the early '90s that Ho, then a virologist at UCLA, heard a high-ranking chemist at Abbott Pharmaceuticals discuss protease inhibitor prototypes. Ho subsequently approached the chemist, Dale Kempf, on an airport check-in line, and told him he had a theory about "how the AIDS virus worked" and how much more ferocious it was than anybody realized. "Dale agreed that maybe we could help each other," Ho later told *the Wall Street Journal.*

By 1993, Abbott had narrowed its hundreds of prospective compounds down to one, which later became the most toxic of the licensed protease inhibitors, Norvir. Meanwhile, philanthropist Irene Diamond had fulfilled her late husband Aaron Diamond's wish to set up a lavish research lab which would attract some of the best scientists in the country. "Irene wanted a star," is how Dr. Steven Miles described it. She chose the quiet, diminutive David Ho to be the director of the Aaron Diamond AIDS Research Center immediately after meeting him and hearing about his research. Ho and his colleagues at Aaron Diamond, Dr. Marty Markowitz, began experimenting with a handful of patients. They gave them the cocktail therapy, measured their drug-resistant mutations, and then calculated "how many virus particles were churned out each day by infected cells," according to Michael Waldholz, reporting in the *Wall Street Journal*. These calculations led to the infamous math model.

The problem is not restricted to the math model, however—the very technique that Ho and Markowitz used to measure and calculate these "virus particles," is itself deeply problematic. Is "viral load" really measuring the amount of virus in one's body? Not according to some of the scientists who have studied the matter closely. As Harvey Bialy notes, "The only important question in AIDS is how much infectious virus there is.... Despite all the noise about massive viremia [levels of virus] and math models coming in from David Ho, the figures remain precisely as Peter Duesberg published in 1987 when he first critiqued the hypothesis.... Only one in 100 T-cells are ever infected, only one in 1,000 are ever making viral proteins, and that corresponds to a tiny amount of virus present in the blood. Everything else is effectively neutralized by the immune system.

"A viral load of 100,000 corresponds to one or less virus particles, which is the only medically relevant barometer. That is not enough to do anything. In the *Nature* paper, Ho manipulated the picture by using PCR and passed it off as infectious virus. When I read it, I said, 'This is fucking nonsense! How do you pass off a biochemical unit as an infectious particle? This will never fly. But it flew.'"

Dr. David Rasnick, who once worked in diagnostics at Abbott, concurs with this view. "'Viral load' is the most powerful microscope ever developed," he says. "If the only way you can see something is by using the most powerful microscope, how clinically relevant can it be? If a person had real viremia you wouldn't need PCR to see it. Here you're talking about a level of about one virus particle in a drop of blood!

"Here's an example. When they look for HIV in breast milk, they do forty-five cycles of PCR, which is a 35-trillion-fold amplification, in order to find enough genetic material. We are at the level of sensitivity of nuclear physics now with this PCR stuff. And David Ho talks about making HIV 'undetectable?' It starts out undetectable. That's the whole point. HIV has always been more or less undetectable.

"So they've taken a number that is next to nothing, and mass multiplied it. But it's still next to nothing. Just a bunch of numbers that are used to scare people and make people go on these drugs.... All this stuff about wanting to get to zero, or to undetectable, is absurd because it implies that a single particle of HIV is lethal, but it's not."

"This is the biological equivalent of counting bumpers in a junkyard and saying they represent functional cars."

In the summer of 1996, thousands of people at the International AIDS Conference in Vancouver listened to Ho's findings from TV monitors hanging through the vast conference halls. The audience listened with rapt attention as Ho revealed his data: Nine patients, he said, who had been on a combination of drugs including some of the new protease inhibitors, had "no evidence of the virus in their bloodstream," after being on the drugs for between ninety and 300 days. Ho calmly repeated his mantra: Because of the new drugs, it was "time to hit HIV, early and hard."

"It was just unadulterated hype. It was preposterous," recalls Dr. Steven Miles, professor of medicine, University of Minnesota Medical School. "It was almost like an instantaneous religion, or a cult, right after Vancouver. You were either a part of that hit-hard-hit-early religion or you were not. It split the HIV community."

But Ho's mathematical model, which "demonstrated" that the virus was "furiously replicating," made the virus suddenly seem more lethal than ever, and in the fervor that followed, doctors who advocated being careful and conservative with drug regimens were seen as foolish pacifists, willfully surrendering to a vicious enemy. A kind of collective fantasy formed in the hushed room at the Vancouver conference, as the low-key scientist unveiled his data, never altering his blank facial expression, but inspiring a mania with his quiet use of a few new buzzwords: "eradication," "undetectable." The idea was that the new drugs could eradicate HIV—get rid of it—and that once it was gone, people could stop taking the drugs and live AIDS-free for the rest of their lives. All agreed that these drugs were not designed for long term use, that they were way too toxic.

Ho cast a powerful spell over not just his audience, but the world's media, medical community, and AIDS community. The excitement that emanated from Ho's presentation was palpable—it spread like wildfire through the media. Within hours, people were rushing in to their doctors' offices, begging for prescriptions. Most of them were healthy. None of them cared about anything except the new magic word: eradication. "It's not even really a mathematical model," says Mark Craddock, a mathematician at the University of Technology-Sydney, referring to Ho's construct. "In my opinion, it's mathematical junk."

Craddock has written several critiques of Ho's model, and says he cannot comprehend how it was ever able to gain such momentum. "Ho's equations predict that over the course of ten years, an HIV-positive person will produce more particles of HIV than there are atoms in the universe. There is no way you could make that much virus."

Mathematical modeling of diseases is a whole area of research unto itself. "It is widely acknowledged in the mathematical biology community," says Craddock, "that AIDS has been damn near impossible to mathematically model properly. No one has succeeded in producing a model that even looks right.... The history of mathematics is full of things that looked right but turned out to be wrong. That is why we insist on proof. You have to check every single detail and make sure it is right. We send a Voyager spacecraft out, and it arrives within a few minutes of predictions at the planet Neptune twenty years after it departed. That is because Newton's theory of gravitation works."

An editorial in the February 1998 issue of *Nature Medicine* by renowned virologist Mario Roederer pointed out that cocktail therapy does not cause T-cells to increase, but rather to be redistributed throughout the body—which is not an immunological advantage. This had been discovered a year earlier when an American group of researchers developed a way to "tag" newly synthesized DNA and isolate T-cell populations. What they found does not bode well for those who are on cocktail drugs: Of three groups—uninfected people, untreated HIV-positive people, and HIV-positive people on the drug—the T-cells of those on the drugs survived the shortest amount of time.

"You don't have to waste a lot of time on this," says Harvey Bialy when I ask him about how and when Ho's research was refuted in the scientific literature. "The Roederer piece finished it. Ho is finished. In the scientific world right now it is firmly established that the model is nonsense." One AIDS researcher and physician who spoke only on condition of anonymity had this to say about Ho's theory: "Everybody in the scientific community has known for years that his HIV model was ludicrously wrong. I remember being at a conference in Chicago two years ago, and Ho's data was shot to shreds by one speaker after another. David Ho got up to speak at the end and there was really nothing he could say."

AIDS physician and researcher Joe Sonnabend scowls when I ask about Ho's math model. "Of course it's wrong," he says impatiently. "Everybody knows that. It's such way-out bullshit. The notion of 'eradication' is just total science fiction. Every retrovirologist knows this. The RNA of retroviruses turns into DNA and becomes part of us. It's part of our being. You can't ever get rid of it." I told Sonnabend that I had heard from researchers—none of whom would go on the record—that Ho had committed what some were calling, at the very least, spurious research, by withholding a vital finding from the data. In his experiments, Ho had shown that protease inhibitors, by stopping HIV, allowed healthy CD4 cells to flourish. But what he didn't reveal was that CD8 cells—a kind of T-cells which have nothing to do with HIV—also increased.

"Yes, he's a fraud," Sonnabend says, "if a fraud means mediocre interpretations of the dynamics of T-cell changes in response to therapy. But, then, who is the fraud? Anybody is capable of having stupid ideas, but what's unusual is getting them onto the front page of the *New York Times* and *Time*. The real villains are the people in your profession, in my opinion. The journalists. We have traditionally depended on the press to protect us from nonsense like this—not anymore. Now people who have feet of clay become oracles thanks to their publicists and the cooperation of journalists. And the real tragedy is that years have been wasted on this David Ho eradication hype. What he did was unspeakable. To dangle a cure in front of such desperate people is the cruelest thing imaginable."

"I heard from a well-placed source that protease inhibitors were approved by the FDA based on Ho's *Nature* paper," says David Rasnick. "There was certainly no clinical data that they were effective, and to this day there is still none."

The rush to get the new protease inhibitors Ho advocated onto the market caused a near-total disintegration of the FDA drug approval process. Some of the drugs were approved in a matter of weeks, a process that normally takes years. But who was going to complain? Certainly not the recipients of the drugs. They would only complain if the drugs were not approved fast enough. So protease inhibitors were approved on small, short trials, in which results were virtually engineered. Data can be skewed to show anything under such circumstances. Toward the end of 1997, a study from Germany showed that almost half of those taking protease inhibitors had their virus levels increase, not decrease. The authors wrote: "The success seen in controlled studies is not necessarily reflected in everyday practice."

"These damn things were released without proper evaluation or testing," says Rasnick, who now devotes considerable time to warning people about protease inhibitors. "Whenever you give a drug, something that is biologically active, you're going to get some responses. You don't know whether it's going to be good, neutral, or negative. You haven't a clue. That's why previously the

FDA approval process was so laborious. It was to protect people against these unknowns, these toxicities."

A few years before protease inhibitors came onto the market, Rasnick attended a conference where a paper authored by a Dr. Paul Saftig, and published in the journal *EMBO*, was presented. It had no relationship to AIDS, but nonetheless stayed vivid in his memory. It was a so-called "knock-out" experiment, in which scientists totally erase a gene from an animal, and then gauge what effect it has. The gene is erased from either a fertilized or non-fertilized egg then implanted, and then the resulting offspring, if there are any, are studied. "Typically what happens," says Rasnick, "is that either the animals are born with absolutely no difference that you detect, or, you don't get any offspring at all."

But this experiment was highly unusual. In it, scientists removed an aspartyl protease known as cathepsin D—one that all humans have—from a group of mice. The mice were all born normal, and for the first three weeks of their lives, appeared to be thriving. But on the twenty-first day, every last one of them died. Autopsies showed that the mice had starved to death. "Their intestines were completely destroyed," says Rasnick. "Also, they had what the authors called fulminate loss of T-cells and B-cells. In other words, their immune systems were shot.

"That study was a real red flag," says Rasnick. "Cathepsin D is the only protease I know that is absolutely essential for life, so you'd want to stay away from it. I remember thinking to myself at the time, thank God we are not working on aspartyl proteases, or making inhibitors for them." When Rasnick began hearing stories of the chronic diarrhea and wasting syndrome that was among many problems to afflict people on the new protease inhibitors, he had a sinking feeling.

"I said, 'Oh shit, it's happening.' You see, there's always crossover. Even though it's not the target, all of these protease inhibitors also inhibit cathepsin D. The same aspartyl protease that they knocked out in the mice."

"And they're giving people up to seven grams a day of this stuff. I don't see how anybody can survive that in the long run. I'd love to see some post-mortems done on these guys who die on cocktails. I'd like to see what their intestines look like."

Rasnick believes it was a grave mistake for the FDA ever to approve protease inhibitors for human use. "I would pull these protease inhibitors off the market based on the Saftig paper alone."

The meaning of the side effects suffered by patients who have been prescribed Highly Active Antiretroviral Therapy (HAART)—the multi-drug regimen that includes protease inhibitors and is now the standard of care for AIDS patients, including adults, children, and pregnant women—is fiercely contested. There are facts and figures, studies and counter-studies, a virtual blizzard of data that could be arranged to show any number of things. The new AIDS drugs have saved people's lives: That's one piece of truth. But the new AIDS drugs have killed people: This is another piece of truth. The drugs have damaged and deformed some people so badly that although they are alive, they wish they were dead. In the end, everybody who is taking protease inhibitors is contributing to one big medical experiment and no one knows what the outcome will be.

"There is absolutely no question whatsoever that protease inhibitors have helped people," notes Joseph Sonnabend. "But they've probably hurt more people than they've helped. That's why it's complicated. The people for whom benefit has been proven beyond a doubt are really sick people who would have died without them three years ago. But the target population for the drug companies are the healthy people, and those people will almost certainly have their lives shortened by these drugs."

"In my experience, I have seen that those who do not take any of these AIDS drugs are the ones who remain healthy and survive," says German physician Claus Koehnlein, who testified at the December 1999 trial of a Montreal woman who refused to give her HIV-positive children cocktail therapy, and then, in a chilling Orwellian scenario, had them taken from her and placed in a foster home where they were being forced to take the drugs.

Indeed, an entire surveillance system has been put in place to ensure that people stick to the new drugs despite their side effects. There are computer chips embedded in bottle caps that record the date and time of each opening. There are beepers, support groups, buddy systems, observation centers where patients take the drugs while being watched, and even groups of AIDS professionals who infiltrate people's social networks to enlist them to help promote and dispense the drugs. They call it "treatment compliance," and it has largely replaced safe-sex as the core social imperative of the AIDS industry. The goal is to get as many HIV-positive people on the drugs as possible, whether they are sick or healthy, and to keep them on them, through debilitating ill effects, which are dismissed as a small price to pay for the benefit of lowering the amount of virus in the blood.

"I treat the individual symptoms—the whole person, not just the virus. I treat them for whatever they are suffering from, and that's that," notes Claus Koehnlein. "I have not lost a single patient in seven years and I've never used cocktail therapy."

But precisely what it means for a life to be "saved" is complicated, especially when the patient was not sick to begin with. As Koehnlein wryly commented, "If you treat completely healthy people you can claim great therapeutic success."

Healthy people were the primary target of David Ho's eradication campaign. As *Time* enthusiastically exhorted: "HIV-positive patients would have to start taking the drugs immediately after infection, before they realize they're sick." Ho's mantra, "Hit hard, hit early," ushered in a new machismo in AIDS treatment, where people seemed to measure their own self-worth by how long they could endure the devastating drugs.

For the chronically ill, the drugs do seem to have important effects, and it seems correct to say that, at some stages of immune collapse, the drugs have helped and maybe even prevented a slide into death, a response known as the "Lazarus effect" in which people literally rise off their deathbeds. But for patients who have yet to become sick, there is far less consensus about the complex and dangerous drug regimes.

Roberto Giraldo, a doctor and expert in infectious and tropical diseases who travels the world treating AIDS, explains the success of HAART as resulting from its various anti-oxidant, anti-viral, and anti-microbial properties. He also argues that in his experience, severe immune deficiency occurs only where severe depletion of vital nutrients has occurred; reversing the illness starts with restoring those nutrients. "Biochemically speaking, people who are malnourished, whether because they are poor, or because they are drug addicts, suffer from oxidization, and lack vitamins A, B, E, zinc, and selenium. This is true of all AIDS patients I have ever seen," Giraldo notes. "We cannot say that protease inhibitors are useless. In 1996 when they started to use protease inhibitors, there is no doubt that there was a change. Before 1996, all the people who used AZT, they were killed. There was no benefit there. Protease inhibitors—they are also very toxic, but they have benefits—they are antioxidants. No doubt they are poison and in the long run they kill the person, but you need proteases in the process of oxidation. Besides that, these drugs are also antibiotics."

One of the unexpected effects of protease inhibitors seen in recent years was a disruption of the body's fat-distribution mechanisms. This in turn has caused strokes and heart attacks in many patients, at the very moment when the drugs were theoretically "working," meaning so-called surrogate markers (CD4 cells and viral load) were going the right way. The other significant danger of HAART proved to be liver and kidney failure, which, according to a study done at the University of Colorado Health Sciences Center, "surpassed deaths due to advanced HIV" in 2002. In 2005 the *Wall Street Journal* reported that, according to a Danish study, AIDS drug cocktails "may double the risk of heart attacks."

"The vast majority—about 75 percent—of people who go on these drugs are completely healthy," says Dr. Steven Miles. "Large numbers of people are being inappropriately treated with drugs they don't need. And their lives are probably being shortened, yes."

At Lemuel Shattuck Hospital in Boston, Massachusetts, a review was done on every HIV-positive patient who died at the hospital between May 1998 and April 1999, and compared to a group of patients who died in 1991, before drug cocktails were available. Of the twenty-two "post-cocktail" deaths, half died of liver toxicity from the drugs, and two more had liver toxicity listed as a secondary cause. The study concluded that liver toxicity was "now the leading cause of death among HIV-positive patients at our institution."

In other words, at this particular hospital, allegedly life-saving AIDS drugs were killing more AIDS patients than AIDS was.

Hospitals around the country were reporting radical increases in heart attacks, strokes, diabetes, and other complications caused primarily by the drug's interference with the body's natural ability to metabolize fat. This is also causing fat redistribution which leads to humpbacks and huge torsos in men, and gigantic breasts in women. At the same time, fat disappears from the face, arms and legs, rendering patients stick-like.

Holly Melroe, a registered nurse at Regions Hospital in St. Paul, Minnesota, wrote in the *Journal of the Association of Nurses in AIDS Care* in 1999 that the drug therapies "may have a greater life-threatening potential than the disease itself."

As Melroe told me in an interview, "We are hospitalizing more people now for the side effects of the drugs than we are for the infections of AIDS. It's a very complicated situation."

Up to 80 percent of her patients were found to have dangerously high cholesterol levels, she said, which had led to heart attacks in many cases. But when I commented that it seems strange for these drugs to continue to be referred to as "life-saving," Melroe quickly said, "Oh, but they are." The death rate, Melroe claimed, had declined by 80 percent in Minnesota over the previous four years.

In March of 1999, a gathering of the world's leading AIDS researchers convened, as they do each year, at the elite Chemotherapy of AIDS Conference, known as the Gordon Conference, in Ventura, California. Nearly half of the 105 people attending were from within the pharmaceutical industry. David Ho was there, as was Martin Markowitz. Markowitz and Ho received a lot of publicity for their ongoing study of twenty-seven people on HAART. "At last year's conference, I asked Markowitz if his patients on HAART were doing better, the same, or worse while on the drugs," Dr. Rasnick told me. "He didn't say a word. He just stood there. I asked the question three times. This time I decided not to ask. If his patients had been doing well, I'm sure he would have let us all know, especially me." Dr. William Cameron, an MD and consultant to the Canadian FDA, "completely demolished the viral load surrogate marker" as a relevant way to measure health or the success of treatments, according to Rasnick. Cameron used as an example the clinical disaster, never reported in the media, of a drug many people were on years ago called ddI. Over a twelve-week study, the drug worked brilliantly on viral load levels, but shortly thereafter turned out to be virulently toxic, in fact lethally so. At the highly private conference, where no press is allowed and attendees are told not to discuss what they hear, even Ho recanted his central tenant, and said, "Viremia [viral levels] are not predictive of clinical outcome."

"People can have a high viral load and be healthy and have a low viral load and be sick and everything in between," Rasnick explained to me. "These guys will admit this between themselves, they just don't admit it publicly." Rasnick caught up with Cameron after his talk. He recounted the conversation: "He said they're 'living longer' during the era of protease inhibitors, but he said they 'look like hell.' He said they're wasting away and they just look like shit. I said, 'Is that because of the drugs?' And he said 'yes.'"

In a 2004 paper published in the journal *AIDS* it was reported that "all 4 classes of antiretrovirals (ARVs) and all 19 FDA approved ARVs have been directly or indirectly associated with life-threatening events and death." The paper was titled "Grade 4 Events Are as Important as AIDS Events in the Era of HAART," and "Grade 4 Events" referred to "serious or life-threatening events."

The most common causes of grade 4 events (drug toxicities) were "liver related." The greatest risk of death was not an AIDS "event" but a drug induced event—heart attack. And "Our finding is that the rate of grade 4 events is greater than the rate of AIDS events, and that the risk of death associated with these grade 4 events was very high for many events. Thus the incidence of AIDS *fails to capture most of the morbidity experienced by patients with HIV infection prescribed HAART.*" In plain English, once again, AIDS drugs can cause death far more effectively than AIDS itself.

The AIDS magazine *POZ* and others like it are filled with protease inhibitor ads that drastically contrast with the cruel reality. The ads feature muscular, tanned, and beautiful people at the peak of their powers: climbing mountains, sprinting over hurdles, sailing, and generally beaming with life.

I talked to one of the most well-known protease models, Michael Weathers, whose handsome face adorns several billboards across America, and he said that he had not only never taken protease inhibitors, but had never taken any AIDS drugs. He is perfectly healthy thirteen years after learning he was positive. "They have this rule that they have to use HIV-positive models for their AIDS drug ads," Weathers comments, "but they certainly do not use models who are using their drugs. That would hardly make for effective advertising." The side effects listed by the drug companies themselves in their own ads number in the hundreds. The toxic effects are so numerous they have broken them down into categories. Within each of the body's systems, up to fifty specific symptoms are listed.

For one of the drugs, Saquinavir, under "Adverse reactions," are listed: "intracranial hemorrhage leading to death" and "pancreatitis leading to death." Leafing through *POZ*, I read the fine print that follows every protease ad. In each and every one, it states that the drugs have killed people. Yet the accompanying text warns in parental tones about the importance of staying on the drugs no matter what. "Be smart," one ad for the Glaxo drug Combivir advises: "Without your HIV drugs, there's nothing to stop the virus from making billions of copies of itself. Next time you're tempted to skip a dose or two, think again.... HIV drugs should be taken on time, every day. That's the only way known to keep enough of each drug in your blood at all times to fight HIV."

Thinking about protease inhibitors is also tied to the assumption that the drugs have reduced the number of AIDS deaths, but a 1997 study by San Francisco Health Department director Mitch Katz exposes a shocking statistic that would appear to dispel the claim that the cocktails have caused AIDS deaths to plummet. Using stored blood samples and computer analyses, the study, published in the *Journal of AIDS and Human Retrovirology*, concluded that new HIV antibody-positive diagnoses peaked in 1982 in San Francisco—two years before HIV even had a name. In San Francisco, HIV-positive diagnoses during the 1990s remained steady at 500 cases a year.

And on a national level, AIDS deaths began dropping at the end of 1994, at least three years before the drugs hit the market, a fact no one disputes.

How, I ask Joe Sonnabend, could all of this hype take place? How could David Ho be made *Man of The Year*? How could the eradication theory be extolled? How is it possible if David Ho's science is as bankrupt as all this?

Sonnabend pushes his glasses up onto his forehead and looks at me almost quizzically. Then he shrugs slightly.

"He had a really good publicist."

Ho's publicist was a man named David Corkery, from the PR firm Fenton Communications. "We took over to manage the cascade of publicity that ensued after he was made Man of The Year," says Corkery, flatly refusing to discuss the matter any further. Referring to the hype, all he would say was, "David Ho did not create all this." I set off in search of ground zero, a beginning, a place where the tornado started turning. I call people who work on the inside of the AIDS machine. They all speak—angrily, but fearfully—of a pharmaceutical industry that makes its presence felt to reporters, scientists, doctors, and AIDS activists. "It is absolutely extraordinary," says Dr. Miles, who says he has been on various drug companies blacklists for saying negative things about their products. "People don't realize all the myriad ways that doctors benefit from the drug companies.... For example, let's say that drug company A likes the message that Dr. C is talking about, they can give a research grant to Dr. C and because it's listed as a 'research grant,' people will say, 'Oh well, this is above board,' when in fact it's nothing more than a glorified under-the-table payment.... Now, let's say that you are Dr. C, and you have a $250,000 research grant from company A. What is the likelihood that you are going to say anything bad about their drugs? Zero. At best you are going to say nothing."

Miles has felt the heat of this situation personally, being one of the few mainstream AIDS doctors who stood up and resisted the hit-hard-hit-early mania.

"Just go to the U.S. Public Health Service web site. Under federal law they have to disclose who they have taken money from. It's right there. Some of these doctors have taken money from fifteen to twenty different companies. If twenty companies that are in the business of making money for drug treatment are giving you money, can you honestly stand up and say, 'Don't treat!'"

Another man, who for years has worked on the inside of AIDS research, implores me not to print his name, swearing he will be out of a job immediately if I do. "Look at the media, that's where it happens," he said. "Look at those earliest pieces about Ho and the cocktails that ran in the *Wall Street Journal*. They are just pure propaganda, pure drug company puff pieces.... And those reporters won the Pulitzer that year for their AIDS reporting. The pharmaceutical industry exerts a huge influence on scientists and journalists. You have to understand that these AIDS journalists have very close relationships with the drug companies, with their PR people. That affects how things get reported. I mean, they fund everything. They fund all the research, first of all. There is almost no such thing as independent research. All clinical trials are paid for by the drug companies."

He laughs when I express alarm at this. "My God are you naive! Everybody—not just David Ho—the reporters, the doctors, everybody is part of this system. They're all part of the same club, and they all play the same game. They all have the same, big egos.

"And nobody—certainly not the reporters—is going to stand up and wave their finger and say, 'This is all a big horrible machine!' You know why? Because they're all profiting from it.... Every year we go to these AIDS conferences, and all the professional AIDS-sters come in, all pumped up. And this is the moment where everybody gets blown. It's just gross."

"Look," he says, "if it were not for the profit motive, there would be no incentive for drug companies to make drugs. Drugs come from drug companies. They don't come from anywhere else. It's an industry, okay? It's just another industry."

The *New York Times* headline on February 16, 2005, had the sound of a mayday distress signal from a fast-sinking ship. Were the implications less tragic, the headline could also be described as absurd. It read: "FDA to Create Advisory Panel To Warn Patients About Drugs."

Prior to the unbelievable events of 2004, most Americans believed that the singular *purpose* of the FDA was to "warn patients about drugs." Now they were proudly announcing an advisory panel as an appendage, a new innovation. It was like the FAA suddenly announcing it was getting into the aviation safety business. The surreal announcement came on the eve of a three day advisory panel hearing into the safety of pain pills like Celebrex, Bextra, and Vioxx—the latter of which was, by itself, estimated to have killed up to 55,000 Americans from heart attacks and strokes. The Vioxx scandal was the iceberg for the pharma-Titanic, but there were countless others striking the nation's front pages in 2004, and they shared common themes: cooked drug data, suppression or outright liquidation of damning evidence, lack of accountability, and crushing, multi-million dollar marketing campaigns that blinded doctors, scientists, the mass media, and even drug regulators to the truth about hastily approved prescription drugs—that they are often lethal.

Every day brought new horrors to the headlines beginning in the fall and winter of 2004 and continuing unabated through 2005: Drug companies suppressed data showing that anti-depressants caused suicide in teenagers, as well as other violent behaviors in both teens and adults, including homicide; ADD drugs had killed scores of children; high levels of mercury in vaccines had been linked to autism and the data had been repressed; a common heartburn drug had caused at least eighty deaths and hundreds of heart attacks before it was withdrawn from the market; and so on and so forth.

Prior to these revelations, the pharmaceutical industry, the regulatory bureaucracies, and even the media had managed to brand anti-pharma sentiment as "fringe," or somehow uncouth. Anti-modernist. Now suddenly you could pack the White House lawn with mainstream Americans who'd lost husbands, wives, or children to some pharmaceutical disaster, botched vaccine, or sloppily conducted experimental trial. Prior to 2004, there had been no narrative to hang these events on, no sense of a systemic, pervasive wrong. It took a tidal wave of deaths and revelations of Enron-grade data tampering before the winds changed direction, and pharma-alarmism went mainstream.

Congressmen and senators on both sides of the political spectrum started brandishing open disgust toward the industry; whistleblowers from inside both the FDA and NIH cropped up; and parents gave harrowing testimonies before Congress. Even reporters lost their reflexive pharma-apologia and started reporting on the dark side of the Brave New World. "The catastrophe of Vioxx, a pain-reliever estimated to have caused fatal heart attacks in 55,000 people, is only 'a symptom of a broken regulatory system that is currently incapable of preventing further such tragedies,'" said embattled FDA drug safety officer Dr. David Graham, in an article in the *New York Times*.

The FDA advisory hearings, held at a hotel in Gaithersburg, Maryland, was packed with so many people that organizers had to set up an overflow room, "that itself overflowed."

A Federal court judge in New Orleans moved to consolidate hundreds of class action lawsuits against Merck, for the Vioxx deaths, as analysts estimated Merck's total liabilities could run as high as $30 billion. Pharmaceutical stocks fell and fell.

President George W. Bush, meanwhile, made the peculiar move of appointing Dr. Lester Crawford, a longstanding FDA employee, in hopes of plugging up the bursting dam. Sounding like a windblown Mikhail Gorbachev in the late 1980s, trying to appropriate and control the very language of the rebellion, Crawford said: "We are in an era of openness."

Crawford was quoted in the *Times* saying: "Our culture, which has received some criticism in recent months, is not to alarm the public when we get a signal. That era is sort of past. What the public, we think, is demanding, is to know as soon as we know what's going on." The "signal" was a euphemism for deaths that drug companies, aided and abetted by the FDA or the NIH, had systematically covered up. And the bio-medical spin machine even had a term ready that would make a bare minimum of decency sound like an impressive evolution: "transparency."

In mid-February, NIH Director Elias Zerhouni declared a sweeping ban on pharmaceutical and biotech cash flow to all NIH scientists, including patents, which had risen to staggering levels during the nine-year reign of his predecessor, Harold Varmus, who had cut all regulations banning financial conflicts of interest. As the crisis deepened and the façade was torn away, the public saw what lay beneath the avuncular exterior of the NIH. The entire Bethesda colossus of federal institutes as well as all the institutes appointed to oversee them, all their foot soldiers, MDs, scientists, the universities themselves, the boards of directors of medical journals, congressional oversight committees, charities, and health organizations—almost every facet of the biomedical industrial complex was found to have pharma wires protruding from its back.

But in the midst of what pharma-watchers thought was the "Berlin Wall moment" of the pharmaceutical empire, amidst all that talk of openness, transparency, and change, something astonishing happened: The panel appointed by the FDA to advise it on the so called COX-2 painkillers (which include Vioxx) voted to keep them on the market. Ten of the thirty-two panelists were revealed, within days, to have had financial ties with the makers of the drugs they were voting on. The *New York Times* reported that if those ten had not cast their votes, the vote would have swung the other way, pushing drugs such as Bextra and Vioxx off the market forever.

"What we're witnessing, really, is medicine turned on its head," said Vera Hassner Sharav, a veteran pharma watchdog who runs a one-woman organization called the Alliance for Human Research Protection. "The do-no-harm principle is turned upside down. It used to be that manufacturers had to prove that the drug is safe and effective in order for the FDA to give it approval for marketing. Now the drugs get approved very quickly, before anybody knows anything and when they're shown to be harmful we want ironclad proof that in *every case* they're going to be harmful. It's absolute craziness. I don't know how to put it.

"People are expendable. It no longer matters in a purely business sense if tens of thousands die. That's the only logical conclusion one could possibly draw from this."

Those on the left tend to blame most ills on free market capitalism, and those on the right on big government. But the chaos really resulted from the merger of the two, like a failed cross species.

Prior to AIDS, it was considered right and good for the FDA to take up to ten years to check a drug for safety and approve it. In 1986, at the peak of AIDS hysteria, ACT UP scaled the walls of the FDA screaming for drugs and blaming the government for the deaths of their friends. To the pharmaceutical industry, it was a dream come true. An unlikely alliance was formed between AIDS activists and the pharmaceutical industry that looked like discord but was actually a conjoined will and agenda, one that persists to this day: to deregulate the FDA and "fast-track" drugs into the pipeline and onto the market. "Drugs into bodies" became ACT UP's mantra, and they got their wish, starting with AZT, which was approved in a then record-breaking fourteen weeks. The by now voluminously documented evidence that AZT was lethal did nothing to diminish the desire for hastily approved, toxic, unproven HIV drugs, of which there are now twenty-six. One of them—Crixivan—was approved in less than six weeks. Scores more were approved in about twelve weeks. The longest approval time for any of them was 10.9 months—a drug called Trizivir.

"This is the other dirty little secret," says Sharav, quietly. "I don't think they intended it, but the AIDS activists went on a kind of kamikaze assault. I would be fascinated to see the documents and internal memos from the pharmaceutical companies when they realized... hey, look what we've got here. These guys opened the floodgates; they did for the industry what it couldn't do itself.

And what was OK for the AIDS drugs became the standard for almost anything. Everything went on the fast track. It's tragic how the drug industry exploited them, really. The industry got everything out of it. Everything."

In 1992, there were about 98,000 AIDS organizations in the United States. In the UK, at one point, there was one AIDS charity for each HIV-positive person. These organizations sprang up like weeds at the peak of AIDS hysteria, in the early 1980s, but then AIDS failed to spread like the wildfire patterns predicted. Many of the AIDS professionals and organizations dissolved, but many stayed in business and even grew. The ones that are still around today, almost without exception, are funded by the pharmaceutical companies that depend on them for propagating AIDS drugs. Yet remarkably, the old terms persist, and these professionals are still referred to as AIDS activists. Today, these AIDS activists have woven themselves into a tight bond with both the government and the pharmaceutical industry, presenting a united front and speaking with essentially one voice.

All of this means there are staggering amounts of money in AIDS; it is like a global corporation, and what it produces and sells is primarily fear. This phalanx of interconnected interests has little or nothing to do in the West, where AIDS cases are scarce, so the new battlefront of recent years is the Third World, where there seems to be infinite possibilities for expansion.

This history of collaboration stretches back to 1992 when reports first surfaced that the manufacturer of AZT, then Burroughs Wellcome, had contributed large sums of money to key AIDS organizations in the United States. There was nothing inherently sinister about that, one might argue, since it was plausible that Wellcome just wanted to improve its karma and help the afflicted community. But knowing that there was a blazing controversy surrounding AZT—regarding its terrible toxicity, whether or not it did much "good," and the validity of clinical studies—raised eyebrows about the objectivity of the AIDS groups in question.

It turned out that, for years, Wellcome had been giving money to a great number of AIDS organizations, large and small. A Chicago-based AIDS organization, Test Positive Aware Network, received $350,000 from Burroughs Wellcome in 1992, a donation which amounted to half of its budget. The group said it used the money to pay for its newsletter. Project Inform, a leading AIDS organization and information service, got $150,000 from Wellcome to upgrade its computer system. Treatment Action Group (TAG), an offshoot of ACT UP, received $10,000, and ACT UP Golden Gate received $2,000. In 1992, TAG founder Peter Staley noted that, "It's hard to find an AIDS organization that hasn't taken money from Burroughs Wellcome."

Responding to the questions of whether the Wellcome money may have influenced his organization's policies, Project Inform Executive Director Martin Delaney said, "In no case do any of these groups report to Burroughs Wellcome. It is entirely appropriate that we seek funding from the companies that have profited from this epidemic." Delaney stressed, "We've criticized the price of AZT, and the validity of some studies. If Burroughs Wellcome does something stupid and irresponsible, we're going to be out here as loudly and strongly as we were in the past." Burroughs Wellcome spokesman Kathy Bartlett insisted, "We are not influencing information. We are doing this to create a broader distribution of information."

From 1987 to 1992, Wellcome contributed more than $5 million to national and community-based organizations that provide HIV-related services and programs, all the while aggressively promoting AZT for early treatment of HIV infection. A Wellcome press release attributed its donations to the company's "strong commitment to improving health care and a tradition of philanthropy."

One of the most problematic developments in the Wellcome funding debate involved ACT UP. ACT UP was fiercely critical of Burroughs Wellcome and other large pharmaceutical companies, charging that they exploited people with AIDS through exorbitant pricing, among other things. Another complaint was that Wellcome, by virtue of its wealth and power, had clogged up federal research trials with its drugs, to the exclusion of other potentially lifesaving treatments. Although ACT UP did not take significant sums of money directly from Wellcome in the early '90s, it did launch a drive to get pharmaceutical companies to donate to community-based research organizations. On June 30, 1992, a press conference was held at which it was announced that Wellcome had donated $1 million to AmFAR as a result of ACT UP's negotiations. "The members of ACT UP were very divided on this," noted Vic Hernandez, a member of the group, in 1992. "I personally am very concerned about this. Look at where the money is going. AmFAR has a very conservative approach to AIDS treatment and to questions about HIV and AIDS." The deal was negotiated by TAG's Peter Staley, a former ACT UP Treatment and Data Committee member who was also part of the famous group that invaded the Wellcome complex and chained themselves to a radiator to protest the price of AZT in 1989.

Staley created TAG in 1992, which was designed to be leaner, meaner, and more efficient at targeting treatment issues than the unwieldy ACT UP. Eventually, Staley worked his way onto the board of directors of AmFAR. It was as a member of all three groups that Staley—using ACT UP's reputation for political tenacity, TAG's stable relationship with Burroughs Wellcome, and AmFAR's mainstream appeal—managed to bring former adversaries ACT UP and Wellcome together.

At the much discussed June 1992 press conference, Staley, representing ACT UP, said, "ACT UP New York is pleased to announce the successful launching of its campaign to solicit funds from the pharmaceutical industry for the Community-Based Clinical Trials Network (CBCTN). Burroughs Wellcome Co. has agreed to provide $1 million as a leadership grant this year, with the possibility of renewals pending reviews of the progress of the clinical trial program." Staley said that ACT UP had contacted fifty pharmaceutical companies asking them to donate funds, with the goal of raising $5 million in 1992 alone. The majority of ACT UP members voted in favor of the fundraising campaign and saw the move as a step in the right direction—with drug companies putting funds back into the community. Others were concerned and felt that Staley used ACT UP's name without really respecting that the move might compromise—or at least appear to compromise—the group's ideological stance.

The controversy raged for many months, but Staley defended himself of charges of attaching ACT UP's name to what some called "dirty money" by saying at a press conference, "A million dollars for AIDS research is a million dollars for AIDS research." "We are at war and must use desperate measures," he told the *Village Voice.* "If I have to take money from the devil to save my life and the lives of my friends, I'll do it."

Staley was convinced that accepting money from pharmaceutical companies would in no way compromise the activist community's integrity, and that both ACT UP and TAG would remain critical as they had been in the past. "I don't like this deal at all," said Bill Dobbs, a longtime member of ACT UP, "because it blurs the lines, and it will ultimately prevent ACT UP from doing what it does best, which is to be a watchdog. Staley can do whatever he wants with TAG, but the fact is he used ACT UP as a club to beat the drug companies with because they're afraid of ACT UP. I find it absurd that ACT UP should wind up assisting Burroughs Wellcome public-relation efforts, and that's exactly what this is for them."

To ACT UP members like Dobbs, who took ACT UP's democratic ideology very seriously, Staley, for all his good efforts, appeared maddeningly oblivious to the fundamental principles of the group. Staley and his ilk brought a kind of "whatever works" methodology to AIDS activism. And while the majority of ACT UP voted in favor of the move, Dobbs contended that many were not fully aware of what they were voting about. "I don't think most of us knew just what Staley was getting ACT UP into here. When it did become clear, it was too late," Dobbs remembered. It's the age-old dilemma—if you have an urgent cause at hand, do the ends justify the means? Said Dobbs, "People ask me, would you rather this money not be spent at all? To which I respond, why do we have to be put in these situations in the first place?"

As it turned out, much of the AIDS activist community's new financial resources were spent on advocating for the expansion of U.S. government research programs on AIDS. And this advocacy work was, in a large part, successful. AIDS, despite killing far fewer people than other diseases—the CDC estimated that 15,798 people died of AIDS in 2004—controls not a huge portion of the federal research budget but an inexplicably colossal one. By 2005, a total of $170 billion taxpayer dollars had gone into HIV/AIDS, all facets included.

In 2005, the NIH allocation for each patient reported to have AIDS was $3,084. Diabetes kills more people than AIDS and breast cancer—which is diagnosed in approximately one in seven women—combined. And yet the corresponding research allocation for diabetes is a mere $80.

If you look at the NIH by its various branches and the distribution of diseases and funds, its increase in AIDS funding from 1999 to 2005 is greater than the entire budget for every major disease. Of the NIH's twenty branches, each and every one "supports HIV/AIDS related activities, consistent with its individual mission." According to the agency's website, the divisions that are "most heavily concerned with HIV, AIDS, and their sequelae, are the National Institute of Allergies and Infectious Diseases (NIAID) [which runs the Division of AIDS (DAIDS)], the NCI (National Cancer Institute), the National Institute on Drug Abuse (NIDA), the National Institute of Mental Health (NIMH), The National Center For Research Resources (NCRR), and National Heart, Lung and Blood Institute (NHLBI), and finally the National Institute of Child and Human Development (NICHD)." In addition, there is an entire office devoted to AIDS called the OAR (Office of AIDS Research) created in the early 1990s at the demand of the most powerful factions of the AIDS activist movement.

Today, TAG claims to be focusing on "the AIDS research effort, both public and private, the drug development process" and "the world's health care delivery systems." It is known as a very influential force at the Division of AIDS. The main leaders of TAG, Mark Harrington and Greg Gonsalves, are often present in meetings at DAIDS and even, it has been said, dictated policy. TAG makes clear from its annual reports and newsletters that it has extended its AIDS treatment activism to the Third World, and has no qualms about dictating and influencing policies there.

Indeed, despite declines in AIDS cases in the U.S., AIDS activism is booming—more than ever before now that the disease has moved, so to speak, to Africa. But it might also be said that the industry has moved its operations, campaigns, and investments to Africa and Southeast Asia. In South Africa, where the wars over drugs like AZT and nevirapine have caused a fury that has basically pitted the President and the ANC against the medical establishment, the media, and a TAG equivalent, an almost all-white activist group called TAC (Treatment Action Campaign). The TAC is funded by TAG, countless NGOs, and German churches.

International activism by Western AIDS organizations has reached such a fevered pitch that, upon the closest possible inspection, it appears that there is no organic, pure, non-pharma-funded, support of anti-HIV drugs. All of the treatment enthusiasts currently working in Africa seem to be funded by the world's largest pharmaceutical companies. One could write volumes about the strange threads and staggering money trail that leads to Africa, but the best thing to do is to look up the donations recorded by the pharmaceutical companies, who openly admit these donations. Call up any mainstream AIDS website, and you will see that the site has been "made possible by unrestricted grants from Boehringer Ingelheim" and other pharmaceutical companies. "Made possible" is precisely the right phrase. It is not that groups receive pharma funding and then change their views. The AIDS activism and research industry, funded by the pharma giants since day one, is a wholly artificial microcosm that only draws its notions of reality from inside its own closed network.

In 2003, freelance journalist Liam Scheff went undercover and broke a story about children being forcibly treated with powerful AIDS drugs, experimental AIDS vaccines, and other mediations as part of a vast network of pediatric trials that used foster kids from New York City's Administration for Children's Services (ACS). The children were under the auspices of a well-funded "nursing facility" for HIV-positive orphans called Incarnation Children's Center (ICC), a facility located in the Washington Heights neighborhood of New York City. Some children in the trials were as young as three months old. Those who refused, or tried to refuse, the medications had gastronomy tubes inserted into their abdomens, which dispensed the drugs straight into their digestive tracts. It was a new and draconian development in the treatment of "pediatric AIDS"—code for mere HIV antibodies, which do not in reality signal inevitable progression to AIDS.

A 2004 paper in the journal *Pediatric*, titled "Gastronomy Tube Insertion for Improvement of Adherence to Highly Active Antiretroviral Therapy in Pediatric Patients with Human Immunodeficiency Virus," describes seventeen children who had tubes inserted after they refused drugs. "Reasons for non-adherence," the paper states, "include refusal, drug tolerability, and adverse reactions." The authors found that after the tube insertions, for which eight children required general anesthesia, "adherence" to the drug regimens was 100 percent. Making it sound routine, clinical, and rational, gastronomy tubes for children and babies are now simply "GT." "GT placement," the authors wrote, "allowed for the use of more potent antiretroviral drugs, e.g., Ritonavir, which are often unpalatable and difficult to administer to younger children." They also found that there were no significant differences in virologic response (viral load and CD4 counts), but gave no other clues about how the children had fared, health wise, after a year of follow-up. All the study's authors were really looking at was whether "adherence" had been improved, results which one could anticipate from feeding drugs directly into the children's stomachs through a device that they cannot remove.

The U.S. Code of Federal regulations prohibit the use of children who are wards of the state from being subjected to experiments involving "greater than minimal risk," and mandate that each child must have an advocate who fights for the best interests of the child. The Associated Press has reported that of 465 children in the New York City experiments, only 142 had an advocate. ACS—the city's child welfare agency—at first claimed only 76 children were involved in the experiments; eventually it admitted it was 465.

On June 16, 2005, the Associated Press reported that the government—specifically the Department of Health and Human Services' Office for Human Research Protections—had concluded after an investigation that NIH and the Columbia Presbyterian Hospital, which ran the trial, "acted unethically," and that "at least some AIDS drug experiments involving foster children violated federal rules designed to ensure vulnerable youths were protected from the risks of medical research." The London *Observer* later revealed that British drug company GlaxoSmithKline sponsored some of the trials, using children at ICC since 1995 "to test the 'safety and tolerance' of AIDS medications, some of which have potentially dangerous side effects."

Despite breaking federal rules designed to protect human subjects, a number of AIDS activists quickly moved to defend the illegal drug trials. In so doing, these activists revealed tactics common to many—tactics that, in many ways, reproduce ACT UP's original "drugs into bodies" mantra.

Jeanne Bergman is a writer and editor for the AIDS journal of Housing Works, one of the most well-funded of New York City's AIDS organizations. Bergman wrote about the pediatric trials in a widely circulated piece from *Housing Works Update* published in late May of 2005, and again in late June in the

New York alternative newspaper *New York Press*. In the former, Bergman's title was "Denial=Death: Defend Incarnation Children's Center and Access to HIV Treatment," and in it she said what ACS did was "really wonderful. It put kids with HIV/AIDS who had no other home into a cozy, first-rate specialized care facility, where they had access to state-of-the-art combination anti-viral therapy under the expert supervision of a brilliant and compassionate staff. That's not a scandal to be investigated; it's an incredible accomplishment to be celebrated."

"Should children of three, six, or even twelve years get to decide if they will or will not take their medicine?" Bergman asked. "Of course not, particularly when irregular dosing may result in multiply drug-resistant HIV. All responsible parents and caregivers understand that children can't make crucial life and death decisions for themselves, and the law recognizes this fact, too, such that children can neither give nor withhold medical consent. Columbia University ran the clinical trials the only way the kids could get the drugs that kept them alive."

But Bergman went on to refer to the many African American activist groups and state politicians who objected to the situation as "deluded," and called a May 5, 2005, New York City Council Hearing on the matter "bizarre" and "a spasm of misinformed grandstanding from a few City Council members." Bergman was already on record with a milder version of her charges in 1997 in a *New York Times* article by Lynda Richardson that bemoaned the black community's resistance to AIDS drugs in general. Nonetheless, the African Americans quoted in the piece seem remarkably prophetic in retrospect. One HIV-positive woman is quoted as saying, "I'm not taking anything. If it's not broke, don't fix it. Everything is going OK with me."

"Who's better to be a guinea pig than us?" said another, describing AIDS drugs quite accurately as "tearing down your liver," pointing out that long-term tests had not been done, and noting that there seemed to be a great zeal to get blacks and Latinos to take these untested drugs. "Doctors say such attitudes are simplistic," the *Times* reporter wrote, adding that the New York State Health Department "now funnels $25 million annually to minority community organizations" in an effort to "combat the distrust."

Bergman, then a senior policy analyst at Housing Works, is cast in the article as somebody who felt the "challenge in minority neighborhoods was not just to make drugs available, but to build trust." As she put it: "I have been struck by our clients' extraordinary cynicism about the possibility that these drugs could work, and the absolute conviction that like Tuskeegee, the AIDS drugs are part of a giant conspiracy." As Bergman wrote in the *Housing Works Update*: "We must fight back with the truth: HIV causes AIDS. Antiretroviral treatments save lives."

Children's true HIV infection status cannot be known until they are at least eighteen months old, and yet infants as young as three months were given the drugs at ICC. It is not known how many children died during the course of the Incarnation trials because ACS and ICC refused to make public the data. The AP reported, "Some foster children died during the studies, but state or city agencies said they could find no records that any deaths were directly caused by experimental treatments."

I obtained the death certificates of two children known to have died at Incarnation during the course of a four-month stint as a researcher on the documentary "Guinea Pig Kids," based on Liam Scheff's original research. (It aired on the BBC and across Europe but never in the United States.)

One child was eleven at the time of death and the other was two. Each certificate is signed by a physician and states that the deaths were due to "natural causes"—the standard cause provided when there is no autopsy. Thus, I learned that neither the NIH nor a major hospital had performed autopsies on children who had died in the course of a multi-million-dollar clinical trials.

The ICC buries its children at a Catholic mass grave in Hawthorne, New York, called Gates of Heaven Cemetery. The grave is a large hole in the ground covered by Astroturf. According to the cemetery director, the children are not embalmed and their bodies cannot be exhumed. Around the mass grave are six large tombstones in a semi-circle with the names of about 1,000 children engraved along with their dates of birth and death. These are not only ICC children but mostly indigent Catholic babies, children, and even fetuses, whose parents could not afford a proper burial.

I made a list of the names and narrowed it down to the years the ICC experiments were taking place. Then I took those names to the Department of Health's birth/death archives and searched for matches. My colleague on the project, Milena Schwager, had been given some names of children who were rumored to have died during the experiments from foster parents inside ICC. We ended up with the names of a handful of kids who had died at ICC, and I set about trying to find out their cause of death. This is where the trail went cold: Unless an immediate blood relative demands an autopsy, none is done in situations like this and the cause of death is simply listed as "natural."

For two of the dead ICC children, I managed to get a friend of a friend who is a funeral director to send for their death certificates, and he told me in advance to expect them to say "natural causes." The system is designed that way, he said, so that the paperwork moves quickly and the burial happens fast. One father of a dead ICC child was in prison when the boy died. He searched high and low for any information about what had happened to the boy or where he was buried. ICC told him that they were very sorry, but all the medical records had been "destroyed in a warehouse fire" in New Jersey.

Can we say for sure that these children died of the known and potentially lethal toxicities of anti-HIV drugs? No. But the reason we can't know that or say that is that, although the NIH puts about $10 billion per year into HIV research, it as if it has been arranged that all data reach a vanishing point at death.

During the course of my work on the documentary, I located a nurse who worked at a summer camp where her sole job was to administer the drugs to the ICC kids. She was instructed to make sure they got the drugs—no matter what. She told of children screaming, running, scaling walls, charming, and cajoling—anything to be spared the drugs. She concurred with the testimony of Jacqueline Hoerger, who said at the May 5, 2005, City Council hearing that while on the drugs the children were listless, vomiting, unable to walk, but as soon as they go off them "they become children again, right away." Hoerger had her two foster daughters seized on a Saturday morning, while they were still in their pajamas, because authorities learned that she had taken them off the drugs. They became healthy right away when she did so, but she nonethless lost all visitation rights and does not know what has since happened to the two girls she loved and wanted to adopt.

The nurse who came forward anonymously to me said that all the ICC kids spent the entire ten-day camp stay in the infirmary, lying in beds, lifeless. She said she had been told the drugs were in the best interests of the kids, but she decided to speak out because she knew "something was wrong."

The New York City Council Hearing about the ICC affair was packed and the air was electric. It felt like an historic event. ACS Commissioner John Mattingly started out by making the mistake of calling those who were furious about the trials "fringe groups" and was put in his place, as though by the swipe of a mighty lion paw, by Councilman Bill Perkins who said in a low, rich voice: "An apology is in order, I believe, for your use of this phrase 'fringe groups.' To use that phrase diminishes the substance of what we are talking about. There is nothing of greater concern to communities of color than what we are talking about here today. This has grave racial and historical connotations, and you, sir, have opened a real can of worms." The audience roared. After Perkins' statement, Mattingly was contrite, vowing to "find out what happened to these children. Every one of them."

Public Advocate Dr. Betsy Gotbaum, whose inquiries to ACS and ICC about details of the trials had gone unanswered, said: "This is so outrageous. It is literally unbelievable."

The meeting went on for about five hours, concluding with three-minute testimonies from dozens of people, including parents whose children had been taken into custody by ACS and made part of the medical experiments. Many people cried openly.

What happened at ICC, we must conclude, was most certainly a scandal. But the most revealing part of the story is the speed that AIDS activists responded to criticism of the ICC trials. Before the facts of the case could be known—before critics, politicians, or journalists knew the full story—AIDS activists responded with uncritical support. As if a pharma-think had overtaken their work, the possibility of misconduct was never seriously considered. Research must go forward, they insisted. And treatment must go on.

Joyce Ann Hafford was a single mother living alone with her thirteen-year-old son, Jermal, in Memphis, Tennessee, when she learned that she was pregnant with her second child. She worked as a customer service representative at a company called CMC Call Center; her son was a top student, an athlete and musician. In April 2003, Hafford, four months pregnant, was urged by her obstetrician to take an HIV test. She agreed, even though she was healthy and had no reason to think she might be HIV-positive. The test result came up positive, though Hafford was tested only once, and she did not know that pregnancy itself can cause a false positive HIV test. Her first thought was of her unborn baby. Hafford was immediately referred to an HIV/AIDS specialist, Dr. Edwin Thorpe, who happened to be one of the principal investigators recruiting patients for a clinical trial at the University of Tennessee Medical Group that was sponsored by the Division of AIDS (DAIDS)—the chief branch of HIV/AIDS research within the National Institutes of Health.

The objective of the trial, PACTG 1022, was to compare the "treatment-limiting toxicities" of two anti-HIV drug regimens. The core drugs being compared were nelfinavir (trade name Viracept) and nevirapine (trade name Viramune). To that regimen, in each arm, two more drugs were added—zidovudine (AZT) and lamivudine (Epivir) in a branded combination called Combivir. PACTG 1022 was a "safety" trial as well as an efficacy trial, which means that pregnant women were being used as research subjects to investigate "safety" and yet the trial was probing the outer limits of bearable toxicity. Given the reigning beliefs about HIV's pathogenicity, such trials are fairly commonplace, especially in the post-1994 era, when AZT was hailed for cutting transmission rates from mother to child.

The goal of PACTG 1022 was to recruit at least 440 pregnant women across the nation, of which fifteen were to be enrolled in the University of Tennessee Medical Group. The plan was to assign the study's participants to one of two groups, with each receiving three HIV drugs, starting as early as ten weeks of gestation. Of the four drugs in this study, three belong to the FDA's category "C," which means that safety to either mother or fetus has not been adequately established.

Joyce Ann Hafford was thirty-three years old and had always been healthy. She showed no signs of any of the clinical markers associated with AIDS: Her CD4 counts, which measure the lymphocytes that are used to indicate how strong a person's immune system is, and which HIV is believed to slowly corrode, were in the normal range, and she felt fine. In early June 2003, she was enrolled in the trial and on June 18 took her first doses of the drugs. "She felt very sick right away," recalls her older sister, Rubbie King. "Within seventy-two hours, she had a very bad rash, welts all over her face, hands, and arms. That was the first sign that there was a problem. I told her to call her doctor and she did, but they just told her to put hydrocortisone cream on it. I later learned that a rash is a very bad sign, but they didn't seem alarmed at all."

Hafford was on the drug regimen for thirty-eight days. "Her health started to deteriorate from the moment she went on the drugs," says King. "She was always in pain, constantly throwing up, and finally she got to the point where all she could do was lie down." The sisters kept the news of Hafford's HIV test and of the trial itself from their mother, and Hafford herself attributed her sickness and nausea to being pregnant. She was a cheerful person, not a complainer, and she was convinced that she was lucky to have gotten into this trial. "She said to me, 'Nell'—that's what she called me—'I have got to get through this. I can't let my baby get this virus.' I said, 'Well, I understand that, but you're awful sick.' But she never expressed any fear because she thought this was going to keep her baby from being HIV-positive. She didn't even know she was in trouble."

On July 16, at her scheduled exam, Hafford's doctor took note of the rash, which was "pruritic and macular-papular," and also noted that she was suffering hyperpigmentation, as well as ongoing nausea, pain, and vomiting. By this time all she could keep down were cans of Ensure. Her blood was drawn for lab tests, but she was not taken off the study drugs, according to legal documents and internal NIH memos.

Eight days later, Hafford went to the Regional Medical Center "fully symptomatic," with what legal documents characterize as including: "yellow eyes, thirst, darkening of her arms, tiredness, and nausea without vomiting." She also had a rapid heartbeat and difficulty breathing. Labs were drawn, and she was sent home, still on the drugs. The next day, July 25, Hafford was summoned back to the hospital after her lab reports from nine days earlier were finally reviewed. She was admitted to the hospital's ICU with "acute and subacute necrosis of the liver, secondary to drug toxicity, acute renal failure, anemia, septicemia, premature separation of the placenta," and threatened "premature labor." She was finally taken off the drugs but was already losing consciousness. Hafford's baby, Sterling, was delivered by C-section on July 29, and she remained conscious long enough not to hold him but at least to see him and learn that she'd had a boy. "We joked about it a little, when she was still coming in and out of consciousness in ICU," Rubbie recalls. "I said to her, 'You talked about me so much when you were pregnant that that baby looks just like me.'" Hafford's last words were a request to be put on a breathing tube. "She said she thought a breathing tube might help her," says Rubbie. "That was the last conversation I had with my sister." In the early morning hours of August 1, Rubbie and her mother got a call to come to the hospital, because doctors had lost Hafford's pulse. Jermal was sleeping, and Rubbie woke her own daughter and instructed her not to tell Jermal anything yet. They went to the hospital, and had been there about ten minutes when Joyce Ann died.

Rubbie recalls that the hospital staff said they would clean her up and then let them sit with her. She also remembered a doctor who asked for their home phone numbers and muttered, "You got a lawsuit." (That person has not resurfaced.) They hadn't been sitting with Hafford's body long when a hospital official came in and asked the family whether they wanted an autopsy performed. "We said yes, we sure do," Rubbie says. The hospital official said it would have to be at their expense—at a cost of $3,000. "We said, 'We don't have $3,000.' My sister didn't have any life insurance or anything," says Rubbie. "She had state health care coverage, and we were already worried about how to get the money together to bury her." Consequently, no autopsy was done. There was a liver biopsy, however, which revealed, according to internal communiqués of DAIDS staff, that Hafford had died of liver failure brought on by nevirapine toxicity.

And what was the family told about the cause of Hafford's death? "How did they put it?" Rubbie answers, carefully. "They told us how safe the drug was, they never attributed her death to the drug itself, at all. They said that her disease, AIDS, must have progressed rapidly." But Joyce Ann Hafford never had AIDS, or anything even on the diagnostic scale of AIDS. "I told my mom when we were walking out of there that morning," Rubbie recalls, "I said, 'Something is wrong.' She said, 'What do you mean?' I said, 'On the one hand they're telling us this drug is so safe, on the other hand they're telling us they're going to monitor the other patients more closely. If her disease was progressing, they could have changed the medication.' I knew something was wrong with their story, but I just could not put my finger on what it was."

When they got home that morning, they broke the news to Jermal. "I think he cried the whole day when we told him," Rubbie recalls. "My mom had tried to prepare him. She said, 'You know, Jermal, my mom died when I was very young,' but he was just devastated. They were like two peas in a pod those two. You could never separate them." Later on, Jermal became consumed with worry about how they would bury his mother, for which they had no funds and no insurance. The community pitched in, and Joyce Ann Hafford was buried. "I haven't even been able to go back to her grave since she passed," says Rubbie.

Rubbie King is haunted by many questions, including whether her sister was really infected with HIV, and also what the long-term damage might be to Sterling, whom Rubbie is now raising, along with Jermal and her own child. Sterling, in addition to the drugs he was exposed to in the womb, was also on an eight-week AZT regimen after birth. One of the reasons the family suspects Hafford may have been a false positive is that St. Jude's Children's Research Hospital has not released Sterling's medical records, and although they have been told that he is now

HIV-negative, they never had any evidence that he was even born positive. (All babies born to an HIV-positive mother will test positive to an HIV test, since they inherit the mother's antibodies, but most will test negative within eighteen months, assuming they are not themselves infected, in which case they start producing their own antibodies.)

Joyce Ann Hafford's family was never told that she died of nevirapine toxicity. "They never said that. We never knew what she had died of until we got the call from [AP reporter] John Solomon, and he sent us the report," says Rubbie King. "It was easier to accept that she died of a lethal disease. That was easier to handle." The family has filed a $10 million lawsuit against the doctors who treated Hafford, the Tennessee Medical Group, St. Jude's Children's Research Hospital, and Boehringer Ingelheim, the drug's manufacturer. Asked to comment about the Hafford case, HIVNET 012, and the larger nevirapine controversy, Boehringer Ingelheim provided the following statement: "Viramune® (nevirapine) was an innovation in anti-HIV treatment as the first member of the nonnucleoside reverse transcriptase inhibitor (NNRTI) class of drugs. Now in its tenth year of use, Viramune has been used as a treatment in more than 800,000 patient-years worldwide."

Rubbie King made a final, disturbing discovery when she was going through her sister's medical records: In addition to discovering that her sister had only ever been given a single HIV test, she also came across the fifteen-page consent form, which was unsigned.

On August 8, 2003, Jonathan Fishbein, who had recently taken a job as the director of the Office for Policy in Clinical Research Operations at DAIDS, wrote an email to his boss, DAIDS director Ed Tramont, alerting him that "there was a fulminant liver failure resulting in death" in a DAIDS trial and that it looked like "nevirapine was the likely culprit." He said that the FDA was being informed. He was referring to Joyce Ann Hafford. Tramont emailed him back, "Ouch. Not much we can do about dumb docs!" This email exchange came to light in December 2004, when AP reporter John Solomon broke the story that Fishbein was seeking whistle-blower protection, in part because he had refused to sign off on the reprimand of an NIH officer who had sent the FDA a safety report concerning the DAIDS trial that launched the worldwide use of nevirapine for pregnant women. The study was called HIVNET 012, and it began in Uganda in 1997.

The internal communiqués from DAIDS around the time of Hafford's death made it clear that doctors knew she had died of nevirapine toxicity. Tramont's reply to Fishbein suggests that he thought blame could he placed squarely with Hafford's doctors, but it was the NIH itself that had conceived of the study as one that tested the "treatment-limiting toxicities" of HIV drugs in pregnant women.

The conclusion of the PACTG 1022 study team was published in the journal *JAIDS* in July of 2004. "The study was suspended," the authors reported, "because of greater than expected toxicity and changes in nevirapine prescribing information." They reported that within the nevirapine group, "one subject developed fulminant hepatic liver failure and died, and another developed Stevens-Johnson syndrome." Stevens-Johnson syndrome is skin necrolysis—a severe toxic reaction that is similar to internal third-degree burns, in which the skin detaches from the body. Another paper, entitled "Toxicity with Continuous Nevirapine in Pregnancy: Results from PACTG 1022," puts the results in charts with artful graphics—a small illustration of Hafford's liver floats in a box, with what looks like a jagged gash running through it. Four of the women in the nevirapine group developed hepatic toxicity.

As Terri Schiavo lay in her fourteenth year of a persistent vegetative state, and the nation erupted into a classically American moral opera over the sanctity of life, Joyce Ann Hafford's story made only a fleeting appearance—accompanied by a photo of her holding a red rose in an article that was also written by the AP's John Solomon. But soon a chorus of condemnation was turned against those who were sensationalizing Hafford's death and the growing HIVNET controversy to condemn nevirapine, which had been branded by the AIDS industry as a "life-saving" drug and a "very important tool" to combat HIV in the Third World.

So-called community AIDS activists were sprung like cuckoo birds from grandfather clocks at the appointed hour to affirm the unwavering AIDS catechism: AIDS drugs save lives. To suggest otherwise is to endanger millions of African babies. Front and center were organizations like the Elizabeth Glaser Pediatric AIDS Foundation, which extolled the importance of nevirapine. Elizabeth Glaser's nevirapine defenders apparently didn't encounter a single media professional who knew, or cared, that the organization had received $1 million from nevirapine's maker, Boehringer Ingelheim, in 2000. "Our mission of eradicating AIDS is always informed and driven by the best available science, not by donations," said Mark Isaac, Elizabeth Glazer's vice president for policy, when asked to comment. "The full body of research, as well as our extensive experience, validates the safety and efficacy of single-dose nevirapine as one of several options to prevent mother-to-child transmission of HIV."

This was no scandal but simply part of a landscape. Pharmaceutical companies fund AIDS organizations, which in turn are quoted uncritically in the media about how many lives their drugs save. This time the AIDS organizations were joined by none other than the White House, which was in the midst of promoting a major program to make nevirapine available across Africa.

Nevirapine had already killed several people. In April of 2000, five South African women died during early clinical trials of nevirapine, while 11 percent of trial subjects suffered liver toxicity. In November of that year, the drug's manufacturer, Boehringer Ingelheim issued a blackbox warning to doctors, citing "Severe, life-threatening and fatal cases of hepatoxicity with Viramune."

All AIDS drugs are toxic, but nevirapine is among the very worst. "It's not a predictable toxicity profile, like the other AIDS drugs. It's more like snake venom. It affects different people very differently," explained Dr. Andrew Maniotis, program Director in the Cell and Developmental Biology of Cancer at the University of Illinois. "The most striking feature of nevirapine is its liver toxicity. It is *extremely* toxic to the liver and organs. And that's why you get the skin necrosis, because the liver isn't the only thing under fire, it's the skin too. You see the nucleside analogue drugs, like AZT, they get into cells and shut down the synthesis of DNA. Nevirapine does more than that. It's supposed to interfere with reverse transcribing of the templates, but there's a lot of protein in the body that it may interact with in addition to the one it is supposedly specific for."

America is a place where people rarely say: Stop. Extreme and unnatural things happen all the time, and nobody seems to know how to hit the brakes. In this muscular, can-do era, we are particularly prone to the seductions of the pharmaceutical industry, which has successfully marketed its ever growing arsenal of drugs as every American's latest right. The buzzword is "access," which has the advantage of short-circuiting the question of whether the drugs actually work, and of obviating the question of whether they are even safe. This situation has had particularly tragic ramifications on the border between the class of Americans with good health insurance, who are essentially consumers of pharmaceutical goods, and those without insurance, some of whom get drugs "free" but with a significant caveat attached: They agree to be experimented on. These people, known in the industry as "recruits," are pulled in via doctors straight from clinics and even recruited on the Internet into the pharmaceutical industry and the government's web of clinical trials, thousands of which have popped up in recent years across the nation and around the world. Such studies help maintain the industry's carefully cultivated image of benign concern, of charity and progress, while at the same time feeding the experimental factories from which new blockbuster drugs emerge. "I call them what they are: human experiments," says Vera Hassner Sharav, of the Alliance for Human Research Protection. "What's happened over the last ten to fifteen years is that profits in medicine shifted from patient care to clinical trials, which is a huge industry now. Everybody involved, except the subject, makes money on it, like a food chain. At the center of it is the NIH, which quietly, while people weren't looking, wound up becoming the partner of industry."

By June 2004, the National Institutes of Health had registered 10,906 clinical trials in ninety countries. The size of these trials, which range from the hundreds to more than 10,000 people for a single study, creates a huge market for trial participants. Participants are motivated by many different factors in different societies but generally by some combination of the promise of better health care, prenatal care, free "access" to drugs, and often—especially in the United States—cash payments. Participating doctors, whose patient-care profits have been dwindling in recent years because of insurance-company restrictions, also add to their incomes by recruiting patients.

When Dr. Jonathan Fishbein got the phone call in January of 2003, inviting him to come work for the NIH, he was immediately intrigued. Having spent his career in "industry," he thought of it as a call to service, a way to do something good in the world.

Over the past decade, as an MD, he'd specialized in the medical safety of clinical trials, rising to become VP of a company called Paraxel International—one of the world's largest "contract research organizations" (CROs)—overseeing clinical trial and drug development for pharmaceutical companies. He had a reputation as one of the world's top authorities on "Good Clinical Practice" (GCP), a set of standards that are collected in a book which Fishbein learned to carry in his briefcase—like a talisman of a lost world. GCP is a set of international standards that were adopted in 1996, as clinical-trial research boomed. During the decade prior to his arrival at DAIDS, Fishbein had overseen and consulted on hundreds of clinical trials for just about every pharmaceutical company. The GCP handbook states: "Compliance with this standard provides public assurance that the rights, safety, and well-being of trial subjects are protected, consistent with the principles that have their origin in the Declaration of Helsinki, and that the clinical trial data are credible."

A Johns Hopkins graduate, and son of a prominent surgeon and attorney, Fishbein had risen swiftly to become one of the nation's most sought-after clinical trials consultants. Crossing over into the public sector was an unusual move for somebody like him. Usually the crossovers went the other way—in the direction of money, i.e., from government *to* industry. It was Jonathan Kagan, the Deputy Director of NIH's troubled Division of AIDS, who called Fishbein and told him not only that he was being wooed for a top position in the division, but that this job was being created for him. The job was to be the director of the newly created Office For Policy in Clinical Research Operations (OPCRO), which fell under DAIDS, which in turn fell under NIAID (National Institute of Allergies and Infectious Diseases) which in turn falls under the larger NIH, which is part of HHS (the U.S. Department of Health and Human Services).

The DAIDS, when Fishbein came to work there in 2003, was running about 400 experimental AIDS drug trials both in the U.S. and abroad, without having any single person whose job focused on "oversight."

"It sounded like a very important position," Fishbein said. "I was to oversee all the staff who conducted all the clinical research operations, both here and abroad." After a series of conversations with Kagan, Fishbein realized that he was, in effect, taking a job that was the equivalent of piloting a plane that was already airborne. "They had all these trials going on, and hundreds of millions of dollars flowing every year, but there was apparently no one there who really had clinical expertise—who knew all the nuances, rules, and regulations in the day-to-day running of clinical trials. Every clinical trial has a really incredible, complex choreography. I had been involved with about 430 clinical trials at that point, so I had considerable experience."

Pharmaceutical companies stage most of their clinical trials in the United States, or in Eastern Europe, whereas the NIH, and particularly DAIDS, has its network of trials in the Third World—primarily in Africa, India, and Asia. Apparently, no one was charged with overseeing them all. The culture shock for Fishbein was to discover that industry, in many ways, has higher standards than the government when it comes to the conduct of clinical trials. Or perhaps more accurately, the government has more clinical trials in countries where Good Clinical Practice tends to disintegrate.

Fishbein was accustomed to the competitive atmosphere of corporate pharmaceutical culture. "Doing this for industry, you're under enormous time constraints," he noted. "They decide to develop a product and they say, 'This has to be on the market in 2004.' There's a marketing strategy in place because the first on the market gets the biggest share and it's just planning what your revenue stream is going to be down the line. And there's shareholders and there's a stock price...you know. Business."

As soon as he got to DAIDS, Fishbein noticed that the place was run "from the bottom up," as opposed to what he was used to in the corporate world—top down. It seemed to him that nobody ever *did* anything except sit in meetings and complain. Where he came from, you got fired if you didn't produce results. The average drug today is estimated to cost $800 million to develop. The obvious paradox is: How can a drug be permitted to fail when so much has been invested in it? The answer is simple: It can't. It almost never happens.

In 1994, Canadian researchers looked at sixty-nine "trials" of anti-arthritis drugs funded by drug companies, the results of which were all published in prominent medical journals. They found that there was not a single case in which a company funded a study that proved unfavorable to its drug. Another study, in 2003, compared drug trials funded by the drug makers and those independently funded. Not surprisingly, the former was four times more likely to produce a favorable outcome. As Richard Smith, the editor of the *British Medical Journal*, pointed out in a 2004 article in the *Guardian*, the technical quality of drug company trials, ironically, tends to be superior, and the trials are more tightly regulated. He described the work of two campaigners against pharmaceutical fraud, Dave Sackett and Andy Oxman, whose spoof company "HARLOT," stood for: "How to Achieve Positive Results Without Actually Lying to Overcome The Truth." Sackett and Oxman are experts (turned campaigners) in the design and analysis of trials, and they described thirteen true-to-life methods for companies to get the results they want. The outcome, as every insider knows, is built into the very design of the trial, and there are many tried and true ways to do this. In recent years, many medical journals have conceded that were they to reject material based on conflicts of interest, they would literally have nothing to publish. Most have officially scrapped the old conflict of interest rules, and instead ask that MDs simply state their conflicts at the bottom of the articles.

Fishbein was excited about the idea of going to work for the most famous man in AIDS research—NIAID Director Anthony Fauci. Working for government, for Fishbein, was more of a calling than working for what he calls "industry," and Fishbein, like so many professionals around the world, wanted to partake in that increasingly abstract endeavor of "fighting AIDS."

"I saw it as a remarkable opportunity," he says.

Fishbein took notes during his initial conversations with Kagan, and one of the things he wrote down, because it struck him, was that he would have "go-no go" authority on clinical trials.

That meant the authority to stop a trial in its tracks if he saw something alarming. And the officials wooing him were, for their part, being open about what they wanted from him. Ed Tramont was known to repeat "like a mantra," that he wanted to "turn the division into a virtual drug company."

"Tramont said that all the time," says Fishbein. "He was a consultant to Merck for a few years, and he admires them immensely. I guess he didn't follow the Vioxx story."

Fishbein saw his primary role at DAIDS as regulatory, but that wasn't what seemed to inspire his new employers.

"For them it was a real coup to get somebody from industry to jump onboard at a really senior level. They wanted greater efficiency, to get drugs streamlined."

He was hired under an increasingly popular loophole called Title 42 that enables the NIH to lure top-level employees from the private sector and pay them much higher salaries, because they are technically outside of the civil service salary structure. This same loophole leaves such an NIH employee dangling, should they one day wind up as a whistleblower.

Fishbein remembers his very first day on the job, when Ed Tramont ushered him into a room seating about forty-fifty people—the core employees of DAIDS. "As soon as I walked in I just felt...that something was very wrong."

Fishbein knew, before he took the job, that there was a troubled study haunting the whole division. Nobody was supposed to talk about it, but it hung heavy in the air. "Something about Uganda, that's all I knew," he says. There was a trial staged there, a big one, that had been plagued with "problems," and there was also a lot of talk about two particular employees connected to this trial that Fishbein would need to get "in line" and discipline. Soon he discovered just how bad the situation was—that it was something that would utterly define first his new job, and later his entire career. "The HIVNET thing... it hit me like a fire hose when I walked in there." A senior DAIDS official closed the door when she had her first meeting with Fishbein. She had also crossed over from the private sector, and so she and Fishbein spoke the same language. "I'm really frightened about the stuff that goes on here," she told him. "We really need somebody."

The official had been to Kampala as part of a monitoring effort and seen what was going on first hand. She told Fishbein that the division's flagship study in Africa—HIVNET 012—had been so wracked with problems, so lacking in regulatory standards, that she truly feared for the safety of the people enrolled in it. She told Fishbein that the trial investigators were "out of control," and that there was no oversight over them, and nobody with either the inclination or the authority to make them adhere to safety standards. What Fishbein subsequently learned entangled him in a story with eerie echoes of John Le Carre's *Constant Gardener*.

The NIH functions as a kind of governmental scaffolding which oversees, governs, and regulates the interests of U.S. science, at home and abroad, including the dissemination of new drugs. The foot soldiers—those who actually do the work in clinical trials, are the "investigators." Investigators are the academic researchers funded by pharmaceutical companies to carry out clinical trials. They stand to gain enormously if a trial yields a commercially successful drug, in terms of patents, royalties, credit, and prestige. The bigger their names get, the more money they attract from industry to push new drugs through trials. Investigators could be seen as contractors, working under the moral and regulatory umbrella of the U.S. government, but funded by the company whose drugs are being tested. Over the last decade, the NIH, working with pharmaceutical money, had either lost or abandoned its authority over the investigators and taken on a new kind of hybrid role as a governmental business.

A few weeks into Fishbein's new employment, in the summer of 2003, he had a meeting with his top boss, NIAID Director Anthony Fauci. He remembers it vividly. "Half the walls were just shelves of data with these blue cloth binders, row upon row... and the other walls were just covered with pictures of Fauci shaking hands with power. Shaking this president's hand and that president's hand." Fishbein remembers Fauci saying to him in "a very ominous voice: 'Do you know why you're here?'" Kagan had advised Fishbein, in preparation for this meeting to say one thing. "He said, 'Just tell him you're here for the science.'"

Fishbein laughs.

"So what did you say?" I asked him.

"I said, 'I'm here to make sure that the research is done to the highest degree of scientific integrity and to protect the study volunteers.'" Those intentions were to be Fishbein's undoing at the NIH.

For our purposes, the story of nevirapine begins in 1996, when the German pharmaceutical giant Boehringer Ingelheim applied for approval of the drug in Canada. The drug had been in development since the early 1990s, which was a boom time for new HIV drugs. Canada rejected nevirapine twice, once in 1996 and again in 1998, after the drug showed no effect on so-called surrogate markers (HIV viral load and CD4 counts) and was alarmingly toxic. In 1996, in the United States, the FDA nonetheless gave the drug conditional approval so that it could be used in combination with other HIV drugs.

By 1996, Johns Hopkins AIDS researcher Brooks Jackson had already generated major funding from the NIH to stage a large trial for nevirapine in Kampala, Uganda, where the "benevolent dictator" Yoweri Museveni had opened his country to the lucrative promise of AIDS drug research, as well as other kinds of pharmaceutically funded medical research. HIVNET 012, according to its original 1997 protocol, was intended to be a four-arm, Phase III, randomized, placebo-controlled trial.

The study was originally titled "HIVNET 012: A Phase III Placebo-Controlled Trial to Determine the Efficacy of Oral AZT and the Efficacy of Oral Nevirapine for the Prevention of Vertical Transmission of HIV-1 Infection in Pregnant Ugandan Women and Their Neonates." "Randomization" means that people are randomly chosen for one arm of the study or another, a procedure that is supposed to even out the variables that could affect the outcome. "Placebo controls" are the bedrock of drug testing and are the only way to know whether the treatment is effective. Phase I trials involve a small group of people, twenty to eighty, and are focused on safety and side effects. In Phase II trials the drug is given to an expanded cohort, between 100 and 300 people, to further evaluate safety and begin to study effectiveness. Phase III drug trials expand further the number of people enrolled, often to more than 1,000, and are meant to confirm a drug's effectiveness, monitor side effects, and compare it with other treatments commonly used.

A small Phase I trial preceded HIVNET 012 that studied the safety, primarily, of nevirapine in pregnant women, but also looked at efficacy. It was called HIVNET 006, and it enrolled twenty-one pregnant women for initial study. Of twenty-two infants born, four died. There were twelve "serious adverse events" reported. The study also showed that there was no lowering of viral load in the mothers who took the study drug—which is the industry standard for interrupting maternal transmission.

The trial's sole sponsor was listed as the National Institute of Allergy and Infectious Diseases, though one of the investigators was a Boehringer employee. The "sample size" was to be 1,500 HIV-1 infected Ugandan women more than thirty-two weeks pregnant. The four arms they would be divided into were 1) A single dose of 200mg nevirapine at onset of labor and a single 2mg dose to the infant forty-eight to seventy-two hours post-delivery; and 2) a corresponding placebo group; 3) 600mg of AZT at onset of labor and 300mg until delivery, with a 4mg AZT dose for the infant lasting seven days after birth; and 4) a corresponding placebo group. There were to be 500 women in each "active agent" arm and 250 in each placebo arm. The study was to last eighteen months, and its "primary endpoints" were to see how these two regimens would affect rates of HIV transmission from mother to child, and to examine the "proportion of infants who are alive and free of HIV at 18 months of age." Another primary objective was to test the "safety/tolerance" of nevirapine and AZT. HIVNET's architects estimated that more than 4,200 HIV-positive pregnant women would deliver at Mulago hospital each year, allowing them to enroll eighty to eighty-five women per month. Consent forms were to be signed by either the mother or a guardian, by signature or "mark." One of the exclusion criteria was "participation during current pregnancy in any other therapeutic or vaccine perinatal trial."

Although HIVNET was designed to be a randomized, placebo-controlled, double-blind, Phase III trial of 1,500 mother/infant pairs, it wound up being a no-placebo, neither double- nor even single-blind Phase II trial of 626 mother/infant pairs. Virtually all of the parameters outlined for HIVNET 012 were eventually shifted, amended, or done away with altogether, beginning with perhaps the most important—the placebo controls. By a "Letter of Amendment" dated March 9, 1998, the placebo-control arms of HIVNET were eliminated. The study as reconstituted thus amounted to a simple comparison of AZT and nevirapine.

On September 4, 1999, the *Lancet* published HIVNET's preliminary results, reporting that "Nevirapine lowered the risk of HIV-I transmission during the first fourteen–sixteen weeks of life by nearly 50 percent." The report concluded that "the two regimens were well-tolerated and adverse events were similar in the two groups." The article also reported that thirty-eight babies had died, sixteen in the nevirapine group and twenty-two in the AZT group. The rate of HIV transmission in the AZT arm was 25 percent, while in the nevirapine group it was only 13 percent. As *Hopkins Medical News* later reported, the study was received rapturously. "The data proved stunning. It showed that nevirapine was 47 percent more effective than AZT and had reduced the number of infected infants from 25 to 13 percent. Best of all, nevirapine was inexpensive—just $4 for both doses. If implemented widely, the drug could prevent HIV transmission in more than 300,000 new-borns a year."

With the results of the study now published in the *Lancet*, Boehringer, which previously had shown little interest in HIVNET, now pressed for FDA approval to have nevirapine licensed for use in preventing the transmission of HIV in pregnancy.

There were complications, however. On December 6, 2000, a research letter in the *Journal of the American Medical Association* warned against using nevirapine for post-exposure treatment after two cases of life-threatening liver toxicity were reported among health-care workers who'd taken the drug for only a few days. (One of them required a liver transplant.) The January 5, 2001, issue of the CDC's *Morbidity and Mortality Weekly Report* (*MMWR*) contained an FDA review of MedWatch—an informal reporting system of drug reactions—that highlighted an additional twenty cases of "serious adverse events" resulting from fairly brief nevirapine post-exposure prophylaxis. "Serious adverse events" (SAE) were defined as anything "life-threatening, permanently disabling," or requiring "prolonged hospitalization, or [...] intervention to prevent permanent impairment or damage." The *MMWR* stressed that there probably were more unreported cases, since the reporting by doctors to MedWatch is "voluntary" and "passive."

But NIAID was on another track altogether, either oblivious of or undeterred by the toxicity controversy. In 2001, Boehringer Ingelheim submitted its supplemental licensing request to the FDA. The request was submitted based entirely on the results of HIVNET, as published in *The Lancet*. Around the same time, the South African Medicines Control Counsel (MCC) conditionally approved nevirapine for experimental use in mother-to-child transmission treatment. To its credit, however, the FDA decided to go to Kampala, inspect the site, and review the data itself.

Since Boehringer had not originally intended to use this study for licensing purposes, it decided to perform its own inspection before the FDA arrived. Boehringer's team arrived in Kampala and did a sample audit. They were the first to discover what shambles the study was. According to Boehringer's pre-inspection report, "serious noncompliance with FDA Regulations was found" in the specific requirements of reporting serious adverse events. Problems also were found in the management of the trial drug and in informed-consent procedures. DAIDS then hired a private contractor, a company named Westat, to go to Uganda and do another pre-inspection. This time the findings were even more alarming. One of the main problems was a "loss of critical records." One of two master logs that included follow-up data on adverse events, including deaths, was said to be missing as the result of a flood. The records failed to make clear which mothers had gotten which drug, when they'd gotten it, or even whether they were still alive at various follow-up points after the study. Drugs were given to the wrong babies, documents were altered, and there was infrequent follow-up, even though one third of the mothers were marked "abnormal" in their charts at discharge. The infants that did receive follow-up care were in many cases small and under-weight for their age. "It was thought to be likely that some, perhaps many, of these infants had serious health problems." The Westat auditors looked at a sample of forty-three such infants, and all forty-three had "adverse events" at twelve months. Of these, only eleven were said to be HIV-positive. The HIVNET team had essentially downgraded all serious adverse events several notches on a scale it had created itself to adapt to "local" standards. That downgrade meant, among other things, that even seemingly "life-threatening" events were logged as not serious. Deaths, unless they occurred within a certain time frame at the beginning of the study, were not reported or were listed as "serious adverse events" rather than deaths. In one case, "a still birth was reported as a Grade 3 adverse event for the mother."

As a defense, the HIVNET team often cited ignorance. They told the Westat monitors that they were unaware of safety-reporting regulations, that they'd had no training in Good Clinical Practice, and that they had "never attempted a Phase III trial." The principal investigators and sub-investigators "all acknowledged the findings [of the audit] as generally correct," the Westat report said. "Dr. Guay and Dr. Jackson noted that many ('thousands') of unreported AE's and SAE's occurred.... They acknowledged their use of their own interpretation of 'serious' and of severity." "All agreed" that the principal and sub-investigators "had generally not seen the trial patients," and "all agreed" that in evaluating adverse and serious adverse events "they had relied almost entirely on second or third hand summaries...without attempting to verify accuracy." Westat also discovered that half the HIV-positive infants were also enrolled in a vitamin A trial, which effectively invalidates any data associated with them.

In light of the Westat report, DAIDS and Boehringer asked the FDA for a postponement of its inspection visit. The FDA responded by demanding to see the report immediately. On March 14, 2002, the FDA called a meeting with DAIDS, Boehringer, and the trial investigators. "They reprimanded the whole gang," says Fishbein. "Then they said to Boehringer: Withdraw your application for extended approval, if you want to avoid a public rejection." Boehringer complied with the FDA's demand, though statements put out by NIAID made it sound as if the company had withdrawn the application for FDA approval in a spirit of profound concern for protocol. In South Africa, a few months later, the news focused on the angry chorus of AIDS experts and activists, speaking as one. The South African MCC was reconsidering its approval of nevirapine for pregnant women because of Boehringer's withdrawal and the growing HIVNET controversy. The Associated Press reported that "activists fear the government, notorious for its sluggish response to the AIDS crisis, is pressuring the council to reject nevirapine, and that it could misrepresent the current discussions as proof the drug is toxic. Studies show nevirapine given to HIV-pregnant women during labor and to their newborn babies can reduce HIV transmission by up to 50 percent." The problem with such statements, of course, is that the study in question was precisely the one that established the claim that nevirapine cut HIV transmission.

Two inspections had now declared HIVNET to be a complete mess: Boehringer's own and Westat's, which had been performed in conjunction with DAIDS. But the ways in which the various players were tethered together made it impossible for DAIDS to condemn the study without condemning itself. Laura Guay, lead author of the HIVNET article in the *Lancet,* responded with the following statement: "Several in-depth reviews of the conduct and results of the HIVNET 012 trial as well as the data collected from subsequent trials and PMTCT programs, have substantiated the HIVNET 012 conclusions that Nevirapine is safe and effective in preventing mother-to-child HIV transmission. Nevirapine remains one of the most important tools for the prevention of mother-to-child HIV transmission in the developing world, where there are still hundreds of thousands of HIV-infected pregnant women who do not have access to any HIV testing, antiretroviral therapy, or HIV care at all. For many programs struggling to establish PMTCT programs with limited resources, Nevirapine is often the only option available." But DAIDS was well aware of what had transpired. Family Health International, the NIH contractor originally responsible for monitoring HIVNET 012, contested the Westat report and said that the results of the study had been validated by the NIH and the Institute of Medicine.

According to DAIDS's public version of events, which was dutifully echoed in the AIDS press, the trouble with HIVNET was that it was unfairly assailed by pedantic saboteurs who could not grasp the necessary difference between U.S. safety standards and the more lenient standards for a country like Uganda. Two weeks after the fifty-seven-page Westat report was delivered, the deputy director of NIAID, Dr. John LaMontagne, had set the tone by stating publicly: "There is no question about the validity [of the HIVNET results]... the problems are in the rather arcane requirements in record keeping." DAIDS was so dismissive of the Westat report that Westat's lawyers eventually put officials on notice that they were impugning Westat's reputation.

Meanwhile, as the investigations continued, nevirapine had long since been recommended by the World Health Organization and registered in at least fifty-three countries, and Boehringer had begun shipping boxes of the drug to maternity wards across the developing world. In 2002, President Bush announced a $500 million program to prevent maternal transmission of HIV in which nevirapine therapy would play a major role—despite the fact that the drug has never received FDA approval for this purpose.

In 2003, when Jonathan Fishbein was drawn into the HIVNET saga, the cover-up (for that, ultimately, is what the NIH response had become) was ongoing. In response to the massive failures documented by Boehringer and Westat, DAIDS embarked on a "remonitoring review" in an attempt to validate the study's results. Ordinarily, an outside contractor would be retained for such a complex project, but DAIDS director Tramont made the decision to keep the remonitoring in-house. Drafting the review was a massive undertaking that took months of research, lengthy interviews with the investigators, and painstaking analysis of poorly organized documentation, as the DAIDS team attempted to learn what had actually taken place in Kampala. Even so, Tramont wanted the HIVNET site reopened in time for President Bush's visit to Uganda. In March 2003, Tramont and his staff gathered together the different sections and substantially rewrote the report, especially the safety section, minimizing the toxicities, deaths, and record-keeping problems. The rewritten report concluded that nevirapine was safe and effective for the treatment of mother-to-child transmission of HIV, thus saving HIVNET 012 from the scrapheap of failed scientific studies.

While preparing the safety review section, however, an NIH medical officer named Betsy Smith noticed a pattern of elevated liver counts among some of the babies in the AZT arm. Following FDA regulations, she drafted a safety report documenting this finding and gave it to Mary Anne Luzar, a DAIDS regulatory affairs branch chief. Luzar forwarded the safety report to the FDA. The HIVNET investigators were furious; Tramont, who had previously signed off on the safety report, ordered a new version to be drafted, essentially retracting the previous one, and sent it to the FDA. Smith and Luzar have been forbidden by the NIH to speak to the press about HIVNET. The political stakes were very high: nevirapine was now a major element in the Administration's new $15 billion African AIDS program—on July 11, President Bush even toured the HIVNET site in Kampala, which DAIDS had reopened for the occasion over Fishbein's objections.

By late June 2003, Jonathan Kagan, the deputy director of DAIDS, asked Fishbein to sign off on a reprimand of Luzar for insubordination. Fishbein reviewed the HIVNET documentation and concluded that Luzar had done nothing wrong, that she had simply followed protocol. Fishbein's refusal to go along with Luzar's reprimand amounted to a refusal to participate in the HIVNET

cover-up. In July, Tramont sent an email to all DAIDS staff
instructing them not to speak about HIVNET at all. "HIVNET
012 has been reviewed, remonitored, debated and scrutinized. To do
any more would be beyond reason. It is time to put it behind us and
move on. Henceforth, all questions, issues and inquiries regarding
HIVNET 012 is [*sic*] to be referred to the Director, DAIDS."

What followed, as internal emails and memorandums clearly
show, was a vicious and personal campaign on the part of Kagan and
Tramont to terminate Fishbein's employment. DAIDS officials
wrote emails in which they worried about how to fire him without
creating repercussions for NIAID Director Anthony Fauci, who had
given Fishbein a commendation for his work. The communiqués
took on conspiratorial tones as Tramont led the operation and
mapped out its challenges. On February 23, 2004, Tramont emailed
Kagan: "Jon, Let's start working on this—Tony [Fauci] will not want
anything to come back on us, so we are going to have to have ironclad documentation, no sense of harassment or unfairness and, like
other personnel actions, this is going to take some work. In
Clauswitzian style, we must overwhelm with 'force.' We will prepare
our paper work, then... go from there." The web now included several more NIH/NIAID employees, who weighed in with suggestions
about how best to expel Fishbein without leaving legally damning
fingerprints on the proceedings.

Fishbein spent months trying to get a fair hearing, petitioning
everyone from Elias Zerhouni, the director of the NIH, to
Secretary of Health Tommy Thompson. It was around this time
that Fishbein became a "ghost." Nobody addressed him in the
corridors, in the elevators, in the cafeteria. "There was an active
campaign to humiliate me," he says. "It was as if I had AIDS
in the early days. I was like Tom Hanks in *Philadelphia*. Nobody
would come near me."

In March 2004, Fishbein began seeking whistle-blower protection. He met with congressional staff and attracted enough attention on Capitol Hill to force the NIH to agree to a study by the National Academy's Institute of Medicine (IOM). The terms of that inquiry were skewed from the outset, however, and the nine-member panel decreed that it would not deal with any questions of misconduct. The panel ignored Fishbein's evidence that DAIDS had covered up the study's failures and relied on testimony from the HIVNET investigators and NIH officials. Not surprisingly, it found that HIVNET's conclusions were valid. Six of the nine members on the panel were NIH grant recipients, with yearly grants ranging from $120,000 to almost $2 million. An internal NIH investigation, which was obtained by the Associated Press last summer, vindicated many of Fishbein's charges and concluded that "it is clear that DAIDS is a troubled organization," and that the Fishbein case "is clearly a sketch of a deeper issue." Kagan and Tramont did not return repeated calls for comment. Instead, an NIH spokesman, Dr. Cliff Lane, said that the agency stands by HIVNET 012.

Fishbein dismissed the IOM report as a whitewash. Indeed, the report's conclusions are hard to credit, given the overwhelming evidence uncovered by the Westat investigation and documentation such as the following email, which was sent by Jonathan Kagan to Ed Tramont on June 19, 2003. Tramont was considering HIVNET researchers Jackson and Guay for an award:

Ed—I've been meaning to respond on this—the bit about the award. I think that's a bit over the top. I think that before we start heaping praise on them we should wait to see if the lessons stick. We cannot lose sight of the fact that they screwed up big time. And you bailed their asses

out. I'm all for forgiveness, etc. I'm not for punishing
them. But it would be "over the top" to me, to be
proclaiming them as heroes. Something to think about
before pushing this award thing.…

NIAID has issued a total ban against any employee speaking
to the press about Fishbein's allegations. Instead, they have posted
"Questions and Answers" about the matter on their website. The
first question is: "Is single-dose nevirapine a safe and effective drug
for the prevention of mother-to-infant transmission of HIV?"

Fishbein has said that due to the spectacular failures of the
HIVNET trial, the answer to this question is not yet known. He
believes that ultimately the HIVNET affair is not "about" nevirapine or even AIDS, but about the conduct of the federal government,
which has been entrusted to do research on human beings and to
uphold basic standards of clinical safety and accuracy.

NIAID answers its first question mechanically and predictably:
"Single-dose nevirapine is a safe and effective drug for preventing
mother-to-infant transmission of HIV. This has been proven by
multiple studies, including the HIVNET 012 study conducted
in Uganda."

A short letter published in the March 10, 2005, issue of *Nature*
quietly unpegged the core claim of NIAID and its satellite organizations in the AIDS industry regarding nevirapine's "effectiveness."
Written by Dr. Valendar Turner, the letter read:

> Sir—While raising concerns about "standards of record
> keeping" in the HIVNET 012 trial in Uganda, in your
> News story, "Activists and Researchers rally behind AIDS
> drug for mothers," you overlook a greater flaw. None of

the available evidence for nevirapine comes from a trial in which it was tested against a placebo. Yet, as the study's senior author has said, a placebo is the only way a scientist can assess a drug's effectiveness with scientific certainty.

The HIVNET 012 trial abandoned its placebo group in early 1998 after only 19 of the 645 mothers randomized had been treated, under pressure of complaints that the use of a placebo was unethical.

The HIV transmission rate reported for nevirapine in the HIVNET 012 study was 13.1 percent. However, without antiviral treatments, mother-to-child transmission rates vary from 12 percent to 48 percent. The HIVNET 012 outcome is higher than the 12 percent transmission rate reported in a prospective study of 561 African women given no antiretroviral treatment.

The letter concluded by asking: "On what basis can it be claimed that 'there's nothing that has in any way invalidated the conclusion that single-dose nevirapine is effective for reducing mother-to-child transmission'? Without supporting evidence from a placebo-controlled randomized trial, such statements seem unwarranted." HIVNET claimed to reduce HIV transmission by "nearly 50 percent" by comparing a nevirapine arm to an AZT arm. Turner's letter points out that 561 African women taking no antivirals transmitted HIV at a rate of 12%. Had nevirapine been asked to compete with that placebo group, it would have lost. As it was, there was no placebo group, so HIVNET's results are a statistical trick in which success is measured against another drug and not against a placebo group—the gold standard of clinical trials. The question should not be: Is nevirapine better than AZT, but, is nevirapine better than nothing?

Independent evidence suggests that it is not.

A 1994 study, for example, that gave vitamin A to pregnant HIV-positive mothers in Malawi reported that those with the highest levels of Vitamin A transmitted HIV at a rate of only 7.2 percent. This is consistent with a vast body of research linking nutritional status to sero-conversion, as well as to general health. Another study on the efficacy of nevirapine in mother-to-child transmission was performed by researchers from Ghent University (Belgium) in Kenya and published in 2004.

Dr. Ann Quaghebeur, who led the Ghent study, was reached at her home near London. I asked her what she thought of the reaction to HIVNET 012. She replied in a very quiet voice, almost a whisper. "Our results showed that nevirapine had little effect. I actually felt it was a waste of resources. HIVNET was just one study, but usually before you apply it in a field setting there should be a few more studies to see if it works in real life. What I think they should have done is wait for more studies before they launched this in all those countries." When I asked her how she explained this, she replied, "Well, I want to be careful, there seems to be an industry now."

The failure of the HIVNET researchers to properly control their study with a placebo group is not as unusual as one might think. In fact, as has been recounted in previous chapters, this failure is perhaps the outstanding characteristic of AIDS research in general. The 1986 Phase II trial that preceded the FDA's approval of AZT was presented as a double-blind, placebo-controlled study, though it was anything but that. As became clear afterward through the efforts of a few journalists, as well as the testimony of participants, the trial was "unblinded" almost immediately because of the severe toxicity of the drug. Members of the control group began to acquire AZT independently or from other study participants, and eventually the study was aborted and everyone was put on the drug. As in the case of HIVNET, documents obtained by *New York Native* reporter John Lauritsen under the Freedom of Information Act subsequently suggested that data-tampering was widespread. Documents were altered, causes of death were unverified, and the researchers tended to assume what they wished to prove, i.e., that placebo-group diseases were AIDS-related but that those in the AZT group were not. So serious were the deviations from experimental protocol at one Boston hospital that an FDA inspector attempted to exclude data from that center. AZT was, of course, approved in record time, but that record didn't stand for long. In 1991, the FDA approved another DNA chain terminator, ddI, without even the pretense of a controlled study. Anti-HIV drugs such as Crixivan were approved in as little as six weeks, and cast as a triumph of AIDS activism. This pattern of jettisoning standard experimental controls has continued up to the present, as the HIVNET affair amply demonstrates, and has characterized not only research into new drugs designed to exterminate HIV but the more fundamental questions at the root of AIDS research.

The HIVNET cover-up, however, can only be understood within the larger political context of AIDS. Its emergence in the 1980s sparked a medical state of emergency in which scientific controls, the rules that are supposed to bracket the emotions and desires of individual researchers, were frequently compromised or removed entirely. As AIDS grew in the 1980s into a global, multibillion-dollar juggernaut of diagnostics, drugs, and activist organizations, it helped turn disease into politics, and politics, at least in the United States, is all about turning power into money.

The nevirapine debate follows the same histrionic, antiscientific pattern. Because he voiced his concerns about the toxicity of this and other antiretroviral drugs, President Thabo Mbeki of South Africa was pilloried in the international press as pharmaceutical companies and their well-funded "activist" ambassadors repeated their mantra about "life-saving drugs." So, too, was Jonathan Fishbein, who had never questioned the premise that HIV causes AIDS, but was tarred and feathered for pointing out that the NIH flagship study on nevirapine was a complete disaster. His offense was his failure to fall in line, his failure to understand, in advance of experimental proof, that nevirapine was too important to fail. And on July 1, 2005, the NIH formally fired him.

Though in the end, they failed to silence him. In late December 2005, Fishbein won his case and was retroactively reinstated at the agency, though he won't be returning to DAIDS. He is unable to discuss the terms of his settlement, but he has promised to continue his commitment to research integrity and the protection of human research subjects.

It's too late to save people like Joyce Ann Hafford, but it is possible that an open and honest debate about the risks of current AIDS treatments and the scientific questions concerning HIV could save others.

The battleground for the war on AIDS is the human body; those who advocate conventional AIDS drug regimens share a belief that any degree of destruction to the human body is still preferable to allowing the virus to go unchecked. It is the virus, and the virus alone, that is the "enemy." In AIDS, as in military wars, death is ennobled by the necessity of battle, the virulence of the enemy. The now twenty-six drugs, in four classes, that have been marketed to tackle the elusive, endlessly cunning virus are described as the *armamentarium* in this war. In addition, there are at least thirty drugs that have been developed to offset the side effects of anti-HIV drugs.

The hysteria-laden question of whether anti-HIV drugs are "life-saving," as the AIDS orthodoxy holds, or "deadly," as the HIV dissidents claim, is unanswerable in the currently available language, which was blunted and rendered incoherent by political forces as early as 1981. Language is the only interface between phenomena and our comprehension of them, and I have grown weary of being forced to use AIDS rhetoric that is itself inaccurate and loaded. First of all, lives can't really be "saved"—they can only be extended. To prove that a life has indeed been extended one must first know, with absolute certainty, that without intervention, the life would have ended. In order to know that, one must know the natural history of the disease, and then one must examine the fate of the untreated population.

But whatever treatments the future might hold, it feels as if we've already been there, and now we need to get back—*back to basic science,* as leading AIDS researchers have been chanting for years. I once pressed the editor of the *Lancet,* a leading British medical journal, to explain exactly what *basic science* might mean. He said that, for one thing, it would mean recognizing that we "have been forced to admit certain things... one of them is that we don't know the true cause of immunodeficiency."

But each nodule of this retrovirus has been spliced and examined in detail, using the most elaborate techniques known to humans. AIDS research has been a dizzying odyssey of high-tech research so elaborate you'd think it *must* be guided by some higher intelligence. And yet nothing happens, year after heartbreaking year. No cure, no vaccine, no nothing. What we have is a vast sea of data—diagnostic tests measuring shadows of cells we never even knew we had—but we still don't know why person A gets sick and person B does not. Official estimates are now saying that at least 5 percent of all HIV-positive people will never develop AIDS. Research is also showing that many people get exposed to HIV but never develop antibodies, because they have a strong enough "cellular immune response" to keep the virus in check. Surely it's worth trying to figure out *why.*

AIDS itself is already a "futuristic" phenomenon in the sense of technology backfiring—casting off a huge cloud of information that tends to obfuscate rather than illuminate. There is also the Orwellian sense of an invasive, if well-intentioned, new social order being imposed that tries to save humanity from itself. But AIDS is so much more than just AIDS. It's so much more than the sum of its parts: its statistics, its death toll, its newly infected. It's so much more than its thirty symptoms, that is, to most of us who live with the luxury of not actually having it. AIDS now has a twenty-five-year history, dense with, above all, death and loss, but also terror, strife and drama, intrigue and hysteria. Hopes, phony cures, violence, fraud, but also incredible acts of compassion and sacrifice.

If the early years of AIDS were characterized by a near-total surrender to the draconian, AZT-centric mandates of the health establishment, we are now entering an era of scientific glasnost. In 1984, a deafening, global alarm went off, warning each and every last one of us that we could be next—that AIDS would wipe out humanity, that the Black Death would seem pale by comparison. Today it has become official that there is no "heterosexual AIDS explosion" in the West. According to original predictions, AIDS was supposed to have decimated, with equal impact, all sections of the population in the U.S., and virtually annihilated Africa. In 1986, Jonathan Mann, then director of the World Health Organization, estimated there would be 100 million HIV infections worldwide by 1990. He was off by over 90 million—in 1990, the WHO said the figure was only eight to ten million. Estimates for the U.S. were also in the millions, and proved to be equally wrong. Gene Antonio—in his terror book *The AIDS Cover-up?*—predicted that 64 million Americans would be dead or dying by the end of 1990.

As AIDS grew in the 1980s into a global, multibillion-dollar juggernaut of diagnostics, drugs, and activist organizations, whose sole target in the fight against AIDS was HIV, something got lost. It is hard to say what exactly, but one can point to loosening standards: Moves away from good clinical practice and the quick approval of untested drugs are some of the most alarming changes we've seen. But the history of the AIDS epidemic has also seen the emergence of an exclusive attitude toward treatment and research where dissent isn't tolerated and the prevailing attitude is that anything goes in the fight against "the virus."

Truth is, AIDS is spreading not along the lines of sexual activity but along economic lines. Poverty in America is now the single greatest "risk factor" for AIDS. In populations where not only drugs, but malnutrition and lack of health care, are problems, we have a perfect setting for the disease. And this of course raises the old question: What *is* AIDS? To what extent is it viral, to what extent associated with living conditions? We have been vastly motivated to explore the viral aspects of AIDS—and all but thoroughly disinterested in exploring the sociological ones.

Which brings me to the core point: The future of AIDS is that it is no longer an equal opportunity sexually transmitted disease but a social catastrophe. Socially disadvantaged women have already been used as guinea pigs (and that is no exaggeration) for very risky experiments such as taking AZT and nevirapine during pregnancy. This is already, in a way, futuristic: Giving carcinogenic and mutagenic drugs to women *while they are pregnant* in the hope of reducing viral transmission by a few percentages.

What next? One AIDS researcher I interviewed in 1995 said, "AIDS won't be perceived as a disease of gay men in twenty years. It will be a disease of impoverished drug addicts and you won't hear much about it." The quick-fix questions—Will there ever be a cure? Will there ever be a vaccine?—are sprung from, and only apply to, other diseases with far simpler causes, like polio or gonorrhea. AIDS, by contrast, has spawned some of the greatest research debates in the history of medicine. Perhaps the single greatest cliché of AIDS is the idea that there is not enough money in it to find a cure. There may be too much money in it to find a cure. And besides, "cure" is the wrong word. "Resolution" is a better one.

But the multi-billion-dollar research agendas die hard. Ultimately, the future of AIDS lies squarely at the feet of a research establishment paralyzed by hubris. If AIDS is ever to be solved, in all its infinite mystery, the very language has to change from the expansionist dogma we've seen so far to a softer, more flexible, less defensive stance. Call it "AIDS research with a human face." Dress it up, tear it down, start over. That's science at its best.

Serious Adverse Events
An Uncensored History of AIDS

		Events			
Year	International	Industrialized world	Developing world	Technology/"best practices"	Epidemiology
1981		U.S. Centers for Disease Control (CDC) issues first warning about occurrence in gay men of rare form of pneumonia that is later determined to be AIDS-related. (1) First reported case of gay-related immunodeficiency disease (GRID) in France. (2) New York Times publishes first news story on AIDS. (1)			
1982		U.S. CDC formally establishes the term "Acquired Immune Deficiency Syndrome (AIDS)." (1) Gay Men's Health Crisis (GMHC) founded in U.S.—first community-based AIDS service provider in U.S. (1)	First AIDS case diagnosed in Brazil. (3) Tuberculosis (TB) is the major cause of death of AIDS patients in Port au Prince, Haiti. (2)		AIDS cases reported from blood transfusions and possible mother-to-child transmission (MTCT). (4) U.S. CDC identifies four risk factors for AIDS: male homosexuality, intravenous drug abuse, Haitian origin, hemophilia A. (1)
1983	Start of global surveillance of AIDS cases by World Health Organization (WHO). (4)		Reports of deaths from "wasting disease" in the Ugandan border village of Lukunya. (2) Peter Piot and officials from the U.S. CDC identify 38 AIDS cases in Kinshasa, Zaire, half of which are women. Results not accepted by journals for a year because reviewers would not believe in heterosexual spread—not published until July 1984 in The Lancet. (2) Unusual patient deaths observed in Lusaka, Zambia, hospitals. (2)	U.S. government issues recommendations for preventing HIV transmission through sexual contact and blood transfusions, including: avoiding sexual contact with persons with AIDS; risk groups refraining from donating plasma and/or blood; evaluating blood screening procedures. (5)	AIDS cases in children incorrectly believed to be from casual household transmission. (4) U.S. CDC adds fifth risk factor: female sexual partners of men with AIDS—suggests general population at risk. (1)

1984	AIDS tabulated as a "notifiable disease" for the first time in U.S. (6)	Zairian government supports establishment of *Projet SIDA* (jointly supported by the Belgian Institute of Tropical Medicine, the U.S. CDC, and the U.S. National Institute of Infectious Diseases) to start a systematic long-term study of HIV/AIDS: HIV infection rate in Kinshasa estimated at 4–8%. (7) Link between HIV and increased TB noted by *Projet SIDA* (Zaïre) researchers. (2) First AIDS case diagnosed in Thailand, among gay men returning from abroad. (8)	Isolation of the human immunodeficiency virus (HIV). (1) U.S. CDC states that abstention from intravenous drug use and reduction of needle-sharing should also be effective in preventing HIV transmission. (1)	13,143 AIDS cases reported worldwide to WHO, cumulatively, from 1979–1984. (9)	
1985	1st International AIDS Conference in Atlanta, Georgia, hosted by U.S. Health and Human Services and WHO. Reports that there was an older AIDS epidemic in Africa that may have originated in monkeys, resulting in blame and "finger-pointing" to Africa as the source of the epidemic. African leaders upset at the insinuation, and resistance develops to foreign researchers. (2)	U.S. blood banks begin screening for HIV. (1) U.S. teen Ryan White is barred from school because he has AIDS; speaks out against stigma and discrimination. (1) U.S. actor Rock Hudson dies from AIDS. (1) Germany distributes 27 million leaflets on AIDS and promotes condom use. (2)	Reported cases of wasting disease ("Juliana's disease") in Kagera, Tanzania. Tanzanian doctors identify these as AIDS cases, based on comparisons with published symptoms in the medical journals in the U.S. AIDS cases are confirmed by Walter Reed Army Hospital among hospital patients (a year earlier) in Lusaka, Zambia.	U.S. government licenses commercial production of first blood test for AIDS. (4) New Bangui definition of AIDS adopted to reflect clinical symptoms. (4) Australian researchers report AIDS case from breastfeeding. (10)	15,202 new AIDS cases worldwide reported to WHO. (9)
1986	U.S. President Reagan first mentions the word "AIDS" in public. (1)	First AIDS cases diagnosed in India and Ethiopia. (11, 12) *Projet SIDA* (Zaïre) finds 1985 infection rate in the general population of Kinshasa is about 1/3 that of gay men in San Francisco. Key	HIV-2, a second strain of HIV, is identified, prevalent in West Africa. (2) U.S. Surgeon General issues report on AIDS calling for education and condom use. (1) Early results of clinical test show AZT (zidovudine) slows down attack of HIV. (13)	28,791 new AIDS cases worldwide reported to WHO. (9)	

Year	International	Events — Industrialized world	Events — Developing world	Technology/"best practices"	Epidemiology
1986 (cont.)			risk factors identified as multiple heterosexual partners, injections with unsterilized needles, and foreign travel. (2)		
1987	WHO-Global Program on AIDS (GPA) established. (1) AIDS is first disease debated on the floor of the United Nations General Assembly. Resolution is passed supporting coordinated response by the UN system. (14) World Health Assembly passes "Global Strategy for the Prevention and Control of AIDS" put forth by GPA, which established the principles of local, national, and international action to prevent and control HIV/AIDS. (2) 81 countries have passed laws against HIV+ people or other social groups at high risk. (2) 3rd International AIDS Conference, Washington, D.C.—U.S. and French researchers denounce discriminatory and irrational policies of the U.S. and governments worldwide. (2)	U.K. Secretary of State for Social Services visits U.S. and shakes hands with an AIDS patient. (4) AIDS Coalition to Unleash Power (ACT UP) founded in U.S.—in response to proposed cost of AZT. (1) Princess Diana opens first AIDS hospital ward and shakes hands with AIDS patients. (4) And the Band Played On: People, Politics and the AIDS Epidemic by Randy Shilts published—details U.S. response to AIDS epidemic. (1) First AIDS case diagnosed in the Soviet Union. (15) U.S. President Reagan made first major speech on AIDS, saying abstinence hasn't been adequately stressed and pointing out that "medicine and morality teach the same lessons." (2)	President Kaunda of Zambia announces his son has died of AIDS. (4) The AIDS Support Organization (TASO) founded in Uganda. (4) Uganda Red Cross begins HIV/AIDS control activities by working alongside rock musician, Philly Lutaya—the first famous Ugandan to go public about his HIV status.	WHO-GPA calls for establishing national AIDS programs in every country and implementing prevention programs including preventing sexual transmission through education, preventing parenteral transmission by keeping blood supplies safe, preventing intravenous drug abuse and educating and treating intravenous drug abusers, ensuring that injecting equipment is sterile, and preventing perinatal transmission. (16) U.S. government approves AZT as the first antiretroviral drug for AIDS treatment. (1)	54,741 new AIDS cases worldwide reported to WHO. (9) WHO-GPA develops modeling software program, Epimodel, to estimate current HIV infections and number of AIDS cases. (17)
1988	World Summit on Ministers of Health meet in London to discuss common AIDS strategy, "endorsed the GPA's 15-point declaration that called for openness and candor between governments and scientists, opposed AIDS-related discrimina-	First comprehensive needle exchange program established in U.S. in Tacoma, Washington. (1) Outbreak of HIV in medical institutions infects over 300 infants in the Kalmykia and Rostov regions of the Soviet Union. (2)	HIV infection rate among IDUs in Bangkok, Thailand, jumps to 40%. (8) HIV infection rate among sex workers in Addis Ababa, Ethiopia, found to be 20%. (8)		75,975 new AIDS cases worldwide reported to WHO. (9)

	tion, gave primacy to national education programs as a means to limit the spread of AIDS, and reaffirmed the GPA's role in international leadership." (2) However, many representatives ignored the message of favoring educational rather than repressive measures to fight the epidemic. First Annual World AIDS Day. (1) GPA increasingly links human rights issues with the spread of HIV/AIDS. (2) Halfdan Mahler resigns as head Director-General of WHO, replaced by Hiroshi Nakajima.	Estimated global external assistance for HIV/AIDS is on the order of $60 million. (18)		
1989	U.S. government creates National Commission on AIDS. (1) AIDS activists stage several major protests about the high costs of AIDS drugs in the U.S. (1)	HIV infection rate among sex workers in Chiang Mai, Thailand, found to be 44%; 0.5% in army conscripts. (8) "100% condom" program among CSWs piloted in one province in Thailand. (8)	WHO issues statement about link between HIV/AIDS and TB, both growing epidemics. (19)	97,243 new AIDS cases worldwide reported to WHO. (9)
1990	Jonathan Mann resigns as head of WHO GPA. (4) Michael Merson replaces Mann. 6th International AIDS Conference in U.S.: NGOs boycott conference to protest U.S. immigration policy. (1) International AIDS Society announces it will not hold conference in country with travel restrictions. (4)	Ryan White dies; U.S. government passes Ryan White Care Act, providing federal funds for community-based care and treatment services. (1)	U.S. government approves AZT for treatment of pediatric AIDS. (1)	102,289 new AIDS cases worldwide reported to WHO. (9)

	Events				
Year	**International**	**Industrialized world**	**Developing world**	**Technology/"best practices"**	**Epidemiology**
1991	WHO sets priority target for prevention: availability of condoms. (4).	U.S. basketball star Magic Johnson announces he is HIV positive. (1)	New Thailand Prime Minister Anand launches AIDS prevention and control program as national priority, including massive public information campaign and national launch of 100% condom program among CSWs. (8) Imperial College (UK) modelers predict that AIDS would generate negative population growth in Africa. (20)	WHO develops guidelines for the clinical management of HIV infection in adults. (21)	125,779 new AIDS cases worldwide reported to WHO. (9)
1992	The World Health Assembly (WHA) endorses WHO's global strategy for prevention and control of AIDS and calls upon member states to: intensify prevention and raise political commitment; adopt the updated global strategy, with particular attention to action directed at women, children and adolescents; integration of AIDS prevention and control with STD activities; improve prevention due to blood and blood products; mobilize national resources for a multisectoral response for prevention and mitigation; adopt measures to oppose discrimination; overcome denial on the scope of the epidemic; and educate health professionals to care for AIDS patients. (22) *AIDS in the World* published. (23)		*AIDS in Africa: Its Present and Future* by Tony Barnett and Piers Blaikie published—predicts grave economic outcomes, dissolution of households and families in Eastern Africa. (25) U.S. State Department releases "White Paper" with predictions of life expectancy at birth reduced by 15 years and infection rates of 10–30% of sub-Saharan Africa. (24)	First successful use of (dual) combination drug therapy. (26) Concern that TB was not only increasing among HIV-positive people, but that this could be raising the risk of acquiring TB in the rest of the population.	149,799 new AIDS cases worldwide reported to WHO. (9)

1993	Russian ballet star Rudolf Nureyev dies from AIDS. (1) Russian government adopts first post-Soviet AIDS legislation. (15) HIV infection rate in army conscripts in Thailand peaks at 4%, after peaking among Northern Thai conscripts the previous year at more than 12%. (8)	Reports of transmission of drug-resistant HIV. (4)		308,353 new AIDS cases worldwide reported to WHO. (9)
1994	The International Conference on Population and Development (ICPD) in Cairo, September 5–13, endorses a plan of action that calls for: (a) reproductive health programs to increase efforts to prevent, detect, and treat STDs; (b) specialized training for health care providers, including family planning providers, for specialized training in prevention, detection, and counseling for STDs, including HIV/AIDS; (c) incorporating information, education, and counseling for responsible sexual behavior and prevention of STDs and HIV into all reproductive health services; and (d) promote reliable supply and distribution of high-quality condoms as integral components of all RH services. "All relevant international organizations, especially the WHO, should significantly increase their procurement." (23)	Condom use among CSWs in Thailand rises to more than 90%, up from 14% in 1988; reported STDs among men decline to about 10% of former levels. (8) Researchers show that the incidence of HIV in Thailand among young army conscripts has declined following increased use of condoms and decline in use of sex workers. (28) Incidence of HIV declines in female Zairian sex workers following targeted condom promotion and STD treatment. (29)	AZT is shown to reduce the risk of mother-to-child transmission of HIV by 67.5 percent. (30) Median time from HIV infection until development of AIDS is measured, drawing on data from homosexual men in hepatitis B vaccine trial cohorts in Amsterdam, New York City, and San Francisco over the period 1978–91: 122 months (10.2 years) from infection until AIDS and 20 months (1.7 years) from initial AIDS diagnosis to death. (31) Median survival time from CD4 T-cell count of 200 among homosexual men in San Francisco increased from 28 months in 1983–86 to 38 months in 1988–93, due primarily to prevention and treatment of pneumocystis carinii pneumonia (PCP). AZT had no effect on survival time. (32) A double-blind randomized controlled trial finds that there's no significant difference in clinical outcome or progression of HIV	152,911 new AIDS cases reported worldwide to WHO. (9)

Year	Events		International	Technology/"best practices"	Epidemiology
	Industrialized world	Developing world			
				disease among HIV positive people treated immediately with AZT and those for whom treatment is deferred. (33) Two-drug anti-retroviral regimens found only moderately effective in reducing morbidity, add less than one year of disease-free survival and have no real benefit on length of life. (34)	
1995		Results of 1995 Demographic and Health Survey in Uganda show reduction in percent of young adults who have ever had sex, increase in condom use, and decline in the percent with a casual partner, which could account for evidence of decline in HIV incidence in Uganda. However, it is not clear whether these changes can be attributed to public policy or the huge toll of AIDS mortality on families in Uganda.	7th International AIDS Conference for PLWHA is held in Durban, South Africa, first time in Africa. (4)	U.S. CDC issues first guidelines on prevention of opportunistic infections (OIs). (1) Results of a randomized controlled trial in Mwanza, Tanzania, find that treatment of symptomatic STDs reduces the incidence of HIV by more than 40%. (35) Researchers present evidence of the impact of harm-reduction programs on maintaining low HIV prevalence among injection drug users. (36) Research suggests treatment should be aggressive and early on in the course of HIV infection, i.e., "hit early, hit hard." (37) U.S. FDA approves first protease inhibitor drug, saquinavir, for treatment of HIV. (38)	WHO estimates 4.7 million new infections; 1.8 million new AIDS cases. (9)
1996	External assistance for HIV/AIDS to low- and middle-income countries	Brazil government begins national ARV distribution. (1)	Joint United Nations Programme on HIV/AIDS (UNAIDS) established	Results from clinical trials show effectiveness of combination ther-	UNAIDS estimates 3 million new infections; 23 million infected as

with 6 co-sponsors (UNDP, UN-ESCO, UNFPA, UNICEF, World Bank, WHO). Peter Piot named head. (1) 11th International AIDS Conference in Vancouver, Canada, highlights effectiveness of HAART. (1) International AIDS Vaccine Initiative (IAVI) founded, launched to accelerate development of preventive AIDS vaccine in developing countries. (1) AIDS in the World I published. (9)

amounts to $300 million. (39)

Short-course AZT is shown effective in preventing mother to child transmission in Africa. (40) Researchers document changes in sexual behavior and a decline in HIV infection among young men in Thailand. (41) Community-based trial of mass treatment of STDs in the population in Rakai, Uganda, finds that STD treatment reduces incidence of STDs but not HIV. (42) These results are diametrically opposite those found in Mwanza, Tanzania, and launch a discussion of conditions under which reduction in conventional STDs will lower HIV incidence.

apy using protease inhibitors, ushering in new era of HAART. (43) Viral load becomes central piece of information for decisions on beginning and modifying treatments. (44)

of the end of 1996 and more than 6 million had already died from AIDS. Total of 30 million have contracted the virus since the beginning of the epidemic. (47)

1997

U.S. CDC reports that U.S. AIDS death rate decreased in 1996. (6)

Domestic spending on AIDS in Thailand peaks at $82 million. (8)

U.S. government issues draft guidelines recommending early, aggressive treatment of HIV-infected individuals with triple-drug therapy—including those who are asymptomatic and otherwise healthy. (45) Annual cost of HAART per patient in Western countries is on the order of $20,000, including drugs, monitoring, outpatient visits. (45) Survival time after HIV infection in developing countries is thought to be less than in the industrialized world—perhaps 7 years—but not much evidence. (46)

UNAIDS reports that as of the end of 1997 (17):
- 5.8 million new infections in that year, of which 590,000 are children under 15
- 30.6 million PLWHA
- 2.3 million deaths from AIDS in that year

| Year | Events | | | | |
	International	Industrialized world	Developing world	Technology/"best practices"	Epidemiology
1998	UNAIDS issues its first report on the Global HIV/AIDS Epidemic. (17) 12th Annual World AIDS Conference, Geneva: Reports of potential problems with HAART, including side effects, treatment adherence, high costs, resistant strains.	14 of the largest donors in OECD/Development Assistance Committee provide $300 million. (18)	Treatment Action Campaign (TAC) forms in South Africa. (1)	Several reports indicate growing signs of treatment failure and side effects from HAART. (1) AZT prices cut 75% after results of MTCT trial in Thailand. (4) AIDSvax starts first large-scale human trial of AIDS vaccine. (4) U.S. CDC issues guidelines suggesting caution in initiating treatment too early. (48)	As of the end of 1998, UNAIDS estimates 5.8 million new infections, of which 590,000 were children under 15; 33.4 million were currently infected worldwide, and 13.9 million died since the beginning of the epidemic. (49)
1999	World AIDS Day focuses on people under 25. (4)		South Africa wins first round in battle with U.S. and pharmaceuticals to force cut in drug prices. (4) Kenyan President Moi declares AIDS a national disaster. (4)	First human vaccine trial begins in developing country, Thailand. (1) Nevirapine found to be more affordable and effective in reducing MTCT. (4)	UNAIDS estimates 34.3 million infected as of the end of 1999, of which 1.3 million are children under 15. 5.4 million new infections in 1999, 2.8 million AIDS deaths, and 18.8 million deaths since the beginning of the epidemic. (18)
2000	Millennium Development Goals announced, including reversing the spread of HIV/AIDS, malaria, and TB. (1) 13th International AIDS Conference is held in South Africa, first time in developing country. (1) UN Security Council meeting held on the issue of AIDS.	U.S. government formally declares AIDS a threat to national security. (1) G8 leaders acknowledge need for additional HIV/AIDS resources. (1) Evidence emerges that HIV incidence is on the rise among gay men in San Francisco and that risk behavior is increasing there and in Sydney, Melbourne, London, New York. (18)	Reports emerge that South African President Mbeki consulted two "dissident" researchers to discuss their views that HIV is not the cause of AIDS. (4) Botswana announces that new contributions from donors will provide ARV therapy for all HIV-infected pregnant women and children. (4)	Disappointing results emerge from nonoxynol-9 studies as microbicide for women. (4)	UNAIDS reports that as of the end of 2000: • 5.3 million new infections • 36.1 million PLWHA • 3.0 million deaths from AIDS in that year. (50)
2001	African Summit in Nigeria calls for tenfold increase in AIDS spending for developing countries—"war chest." (1)		Indian drug company Cipla offers to make AIDS drugs available at reduced prices to Médecins sans Frontières. (4)		UNAIDS reports that as of the end of 2001: • 5.0 million new infections • 40.0 million PLWHA • 3.0 million deaths from AIDS in that year. (51)

Year	Events
2001	Global Fund to Fight AIDS, Tuberculosis, and Malaria (GFATM) established. (4) Stephen Lewis appointed as U.N. Special Envoy for AIDS in Africa. (4) U.N. convenes first ever special General Assembly session on AIDS (UNGASS). (1) 39 pharmaceutical companies withdraw case against South Africa over lower drug prices. (4) Reports emerge from Thailand that new infections are plummeting through widespread condom use.
2002	GFATM receives applications for more than six times the amount anticipated. (4) Available external AIDS assistance to developing countries $1.7 billion. (39) South Africa announces free nevirapine to reduce risk of MTCT. (4) WHO publishes guidelines for providing ARV drugs in resource-poor countries, including list of 12 essential AIDS drugs. (4) UNAIDS reports that as of the end of 2002: • 5.0 million new infections • 42.0 million PLWHA • 3.1 million deaths from AIDS in that year. (53)
2003	WHO declares that the failure to deliver treatment to nearly 6 million people is a global health emergency. (4) WHO announces 3x5 initiative with the goal of providing treatment for 3 million people by 2005 in resource-poor countries. (1) Clinton Foundation secures price reductions for drugs from generic manufacturers. (1) U.S. President Bush proposes spending $15 billion in combating AIDS in Africa and Caribbean over the next five years (PEPFAR). (1) G8 Summit includes special focus on AIDS. (1) Available external assistance for HIV/AIDS in low- and middle-income countries jumps to $4.7 billion. (39) South Africa government announces provision of free ARV drugs in public hospitals. (1) Russian President Putin mentions AIDS in address in Parliament. (15) Chinese Premier Wen shakes hands with AIDS patients for the first time. (52) Vaxgen vaccine trials show no effect on HIV. (4) UNAIDS reduces estimates of PLWHA, citing improved tools, fresh data, and U.N. census information showing some countries in Africa have smaller populations than previously thought. (54) UNAIDS estimates that as of the end of 2003, 38 million (range 35-42 million) people living with HIV/AIDS, 4.8 million newly infected in 2003, and 2.9 million AIDS deaths. Since the beginning of the epidemic, 20 million have died. (39)
2004	Brazil government reaches agreement with pharmaceutical companies to reduce prices of AIDS drugs by one-third. (4) UNAIDS estimates that as of the end of 2004, 39.4 million (range 35.9–44.3 million) are living with HIV/AIDS, 3.1 million died in 2004 (range 2.8–3.5 million) and 4.9 million newly infected in 2004 (range 4.3-6.4 million). (55)

Sources:

1. Kaiser Family Foundation Web site (www.kff.org/hivaids/timeline/).
2. Garrett 1994.
3. OED 2004b.
4. AVERT Web site (www.avert.org/historyi/htm).
5. US CDC, 1983.
6. As reported in Sepkowitz 2001.
7. World Bank 1988 and Zaïre project documents.
8. World Bank 2000e.
9. Mann and Tarantola 1996.
10. Ziegler and others 1985.
11. OED 2003.
12. Vaillancourt and others 2004.
14. UN General Assembly Resolution A/RES/42/8, 26 October 1987.
13. Fischl and others 1987.
15. Twigg and Skolnik 2004.
16. Mann 1987.
17. UNAIDS 1998.
18. UNAIDS 2000a.
19. WHO/GPA, INF/89.4, "Statement on AIDS and Tuberculosis." See also Harries 1989.
20. Anderson and others 1991.
21. WHO, "Guidelines for the clinical management of HIV infection in adults," WHO/GPA/IDS/HCS/91.6, Geneva 1991.
22. Forty-fifth World Health Assembly, Geneva, May 4–14 1992, WHO 45.35, *Global strategy for the prevention and control of AIDS.*
23. *Programme of action of the UN ICPD.* Section on Sexually transmitted diseases and HIV infection, "Actions." http://www.iisd.ca/Cairo/program/p07010.html.
24. Gellman 2000.
25. Barnett and Blaikie 1992.
26. Delta Coordinating Committee 1996.
27. Horner and Moss 1991.

28. Carr and others 1994.
29. Laga and others 1994.
30. Connor and others 1994.
31. Hessol and others 1994.
32. Osmond and others 1994.
33. Concorde Coordinating Committee 1994.
34. As reported in World Bank 2000e.
35. Grosskurth and others 1995.
36. Des Jarlais and others 1995.
37. Ho 1995.
38. Food and Drug Administration, "FDA approves first protease inhibitor drug for treatment of HIV," press release, December 7, 1995.
39. UNAIDS 2004b.
40. Mansergh and others 1996.
41. Nelson and others 1996.
42. Wawer and others 1996.
43. See, for example, National Institutes of Health, "Study Confirms that Combination Treatment Using a Protease Inhibitor Can Delay HIV Disease Progression and Death," press release, February 24, 1997.
44. Mellors and others 1996.
45. World Bank 1997a, p. 179.
46. World Bank 1997a, Box 1.2, p. 21.
47. UNAIDS data, as cited in World Bank 1997a.
48. CDC 1998.
49. UNAIDS 1998.
50. UNAIDS 2000a.
51. UNAIDS 2001a.
52. "Chinese Premier in Landmark Meeting with AIDS Patients," *Agence France-Presse,* December 1, 2003.
53. UNAIDS 2002b.
54. "UN cuts AIDS estimates, but warns pandemic still worsening," *Agence France-Presse,* November 25, 2003.
55. UNAIDS 2004a.

The following timeline, and its accompanying commentary, was composed
by Rodney Richards, a former Amgen employee who worked with Abbott
Laboratories on the development of the ELISA HIV test. It lays out the historical
events leading to the CDC declaring that persons who test positive for antibodies
to HIV are also infected with HIV. Note that "human T-lymphotropic virus
type III," "HTLV-III," "lymphadenopathy-associated virus," "LAV," and
"HIV" are synonymous. Also, other than "*Pneumocystis carinii,*" all italicized
words in the selected quotes below represent Richards' emphasis.

APRIL 1984: DHHS announces the probable cause of AIDS has been found.

MAY 4, 1984: Gallo and colleagues publish four back-to-back articles in
the journal *Science*. One of these papers reports on the "isolation" of virus
from 36% (23/64) of AIDS patients investigated, and from 86% (18/21) of
pre-AIDS patients investigated. (Gallo RC, et al. *Science* 1984; 224: 500-03.)

Comment: Assuming for a moment that the criteria used to declare "isolation"
of HIV in these studies were valid, it is important to note that nearly two-
thirds (64%) of the AIDS patients evaluated in this study had no evidence of
infection with HIV whatsoever. In spite of this observation, the authors
contend this provides "strong evidence of a causative involvement of the virus
in AIDS." This is remarkable, because prior to the publication of these articles,
scientist were reluctant to suggest a causative role for a germ even if it were
found in 100% of patients with a particular illness. Here, a 36% correlation is
held out as "strong evidence" of causality; strong enough for the Department
of Health and Human Services to announce to the global media that the
probable cause of AIDS had been found.

JULY 13, 1984: The CDC comments on the significance of antibody tests
as follows (CDC. "Antibodies to a retrovirus etiologically associated with
acquired immunodeficiency syndrome (AIDS) in populations with increased
incidences of the syndrome." *MMWR* July 13, 1984; 33: 377-9):

"For some, the result may be a false positive caused by infection with an antigenically related virus or nonspecific test factors. The determination of the frequency and cause of falsely positive tests is essential for proper interpretation of test results, but remains to be established, particularly in populations, such as blood donors who belong to no known AIDS risk groups, where the prevalence of true infection with HTLV-III/LAV is expected to be very low."

Regarding the significance of antibodies in those at risk: "A positive test for most individuals in populations at greater risk of acquiring AIDS will probably mean that the individual *has been* infected at some time with HTLV-III/LAV. *Whether the person is currently infected or immune is not known*, based on the serologic test alone..."

And regarding the notion that antibodies equal infection; "... *the frequency of virus in antibody-positive persons is yet to be determined.*"

JANUARY 11, 1985: The CDC comments on the pending FDA approval of Abbott Laboratories ELISA for screening the blood supply (CDC. "Provisional public health services inter-agency recommendations for screening donated blood and plasma for antibody to the virus causing acquired immunodeficiency syndrome." *MMWR* January 11, 1985; 34: 1-5):

"Tests to detect antibody to HTLV-III will be licensed and commercially available in the United States in the near future to screen blood and plasma for laboratory evidence of infection with the virus."

"Persons accepted as donors should be informed that their blood or plasma will be tested for HTLV-III antibody. Persons not wishing to have their blood or plasma tested must refrain from donation. Donors should be told that they will be notified if their test is positive and that they may be placed on the collection facility's donor deferral list..."

"When the ELISA is used to screen populations in whom the prevalence of HTLV-III infection is low, *the proportion of positive results that are falsely positive will be high*. Therefore, the ELISA should be repeated on all seropositive specimens before the donor is notified."

"If the repeat ELISA test is positive or if other tests are positive, it is the responsibility of the collection facility to ensure that the donor is notified." Regarding the significance of a repeatedly positive ELISA: "At present, *the proportion of these seropositive donors who have been infected with HTLV-III is not known.* It is, therefore, important to emphasize to the donor that the positive result is a preliminary finding that may not represent true infection. To determine the significance of a positive test, the donor should be referred to a physician for evaluation."

And even if infected: "*The prognosis for an individual infected with HTLV-III over the long term is not known.*"

MARCH 2, 1985: The FDA approves Abbott's ELISA for blood screening. Among other things, the package insert for this product emphasizes:

"At present there is no recognized standard for establishing the presence or absence of HIV-1 *antibody* in human blood." And: "The risk of an asymptomatic person with a repeatably reactive serum sample developing AIDS or an AIDS-related condition is *not known*."

AUGUST 9, 1985: The CDC reports on the use of ELISA for screening blood, and hints at the possible use of antibody tests for diagnosing infection (CDC. "Update: Public Health Service Workshop on Human T-Lymphotropic Virus Type III Antibody Testing – United States." *MMWR* August 9, 1985; 34: 477-8.)

"The Atlanta Region of the American Red Cross (ARC) and CDC reported data from testing more than 51,000 blood donors, of whom 0.23% were repeatedly reactive by the Abbott EIA method. Among the specimens from 106 blood donors with repeatedly reactive tests, thirty-four (32%) were strongly reactive.... EIA tests categorized as strongly reactive correlated highly with both positive Western blot tests (94%) and culture for HTLV-III/lymphadenopathy-associated virus (LAV) (56%)."

In other words, 44% of blood donors found to be strongly positive for antibodies to HIV had no evidence of virus by culture.

[Note, the full results or this study–along with the notion that antibodies can be used to diagnose infection–would come to be published in July of 1986. See below.]

Regarding high risk individuals: "...virus isolations were attempted from homosexual men attending a clinic for sexually transmitted diseases in San Francisco, California. None of seventy men with negative HTLV-III antibody tests had a positive culture, while forty-three (60%) of seventy-two with repeatedly reactive tests were culture positive."

Or stated conversely, 40% of confirmed antibody positive high-risk individuals had no evidence of virus by culture.

MARCH 14, 1986: The CDC says antibody positive individuals should be *presumed* to be infected (CDC. "Additional recommendations to reduce sexual and drug abuse-related transmission of human T-lymphotropic virus type III/lymphadenopathy-associated virus." *MMWR* March 14, 1986; 35: 152-5).

"Since a large proportion of seropositive asymptomatic persons have been shown to be viremic (5), all seropositive individuals, whether symptomatic or not, must be *presumed* capable of transmitting this infection."

Remarkably, the reference (5) used to justify this statement is the January 11, 1985 CDC publication referred to above which states among other things:

"At present, the proportion of these seropositive donors who have been infected with HTLV-III is not known."

MAY 23, 1986: The CDC again hints that antibody positive individuals should be considered to be infected (CDC. "Current trends classification system for Human T-lymphotropic virus type III/lymphadenopathy-associated virus infections." *MMWR* May 23, 1986; 35(20): 334-9).

"*For public health purposes*, patients with repeatedly reactive screening tests for HTLV-III/LAV *antibody* (e.g., enzyme-linked immunosorbent assay) in whom *antibody* is also identified by the use of supplemental tests (e.g., Western blot, immunofluorescence assay) *should be considered both infected and infective* (8-10)."

References 8-10 are to: 8) The July 13, 1984 CDC report that states, "...*the frequency of virus in antibody-positive persons is yet to be determined*;" 9) The August 9, 1985 CDC report, which makes no mention of whether or not antibody tests should be used to declare infection; and 10) the March 14, 1986 CDC report, which references the January 11, 1985 report that states, "*the proportion of these seropositive donors who have been infected with HTLV-III is not known.*"

Comment: It is important to note that up to this point, study after study has demonstrated that a large proportion of patients considered positive by antibody testing had no evidence of virus by culture (and this further presupposes that the criteria used to call a culture positive for HIV is valid in the first place). So why on earth would the CDC tells us that all such patients should be *considered*, or *presumed* to be infected? Well, it is important to note the distinction, "*for public health purposes*," in the above quote. In other words, what is the proper thing to do with antibody test results if we want to keep the hypothetical HIV from spreading (i.e., further infecting the general public)? Well, given that there may be, lets say a 50-60% chance that persons with positive antibody tests are also "infected" (i.e., they would score positive on culture if it could be done), you have to consider, or presume, all of them to be infected (i.e., sacrifice the individual for the well being of the public).

JULY 18, 1986: Researchers from the CDC publish an article in the *Journal of the American Medical Association (JAMA)*, which *defines* antibodies as equal to infection (Ward JW, et al. "Laboratory and epidemiologic evalustion of an enzyme immunoassay for antibodies to HTLV-III." *JAMA* July 18, 1986; 256: 357-61).

This study is a final report of the data collected on blood donors in Atlanta, which the CDC reported on in their August 9, 1985 report.

Regarding "isolation" of virus from blood donors found to be positive for antibodies (i.e., positive on ELISA and WB), the authors report: "23 (63.9%) of the 36 Western blot-positive specimens cultured for HTLV-III/LAV were positive..."

In other words, no evidence of virus could be found in 36% of "confirmed" antibody positive blood donors.

Regarding the notion of using antibody tests for diagnosing infection, the authors emphasize: "Evaluation of a new test requires an established or known standard for comparison. At this point, however, *no established standard exists for identifying HTLV-III infection in asymptomatic people.*"

How can that be? Citing Gallo's work (*Science* 1984; 224: 500-03), they emphasize, "Current culture methods for HTLV-III identify virus in only 36% to 85% of persons with AIDS or related conditions and *cannot* be used as an absolute standard for HTLV-III/LAV infection."

Comment: The reason these researchers assert that culture *cannot* be used as an absolute standard for the detection of HIV is because it is not telling them what they want to hear. They want 100% of persons with AIDS or related conditions to test positive on culture—a necessary (but not sufficient) requirement to declare a possible causative role between HIV and AIDS. So somehow, they already know HIV is the cause of AIDS, and since culture does not score positive on 100% of these patients, there must be something wrong with the culture.

The authors go on: "For this reason, we *defined* specimens positive on Western blot or culture as positive for infection with HTLV-III/LAV."

In other words, for those samples that don't behave properly (i.e., positive for antibodies, but negative on culture), one must simply *define* them as positive. [Note, five of the six authors on this paper worked at the CDC. Clearly, the CDC is pushing the notion that antibodies equal infection.]

MARCH 19, 1987: FDA approves AZT (Retrovir) for "management of certain adult patients with symptomatic HIV *infection* (AIDS and advanced ARC) who have a history of cytologically confirmed *Pneumocystis carinii* pneumonia (PCP) or an absolute CD4 (T4 helper/inducer) lymphocyte count of less than $200/mm^3$ in the peripheral blood before therapy is begun."

APRIL 30, 1987: FDA approves Western blot "for screening blood and for validating an initial screening of donated blood for *antibodies* to the virus that causes AIDS, acquired immunodeficiency syndrome." "Robert E. Windom, MD, HHS assistant secretary for health, emphasized that individuals with antibody-positive Western blot results should be referred for medical evaluation, which may include additional testing. *The significance of antibodies in an asymptomatic individual* [blood donor] *is not known*" (Susan Cruzan. *FDA News* 4/30/1987; P87-11).

According to the manufacturer of this test (Biotech Research Laboratories, Inc. of Rockville, Md. Marketed by Du Pont de Nemours and Company of Wilmington, Del.), "a Positive result *may* indicate infection with HIV-1." According to the manufacturer of another Western blot, "A sample that is reactive in both the EIA [i.e., ELISA] screening test and the Western blot is *presumed* to be positive for *antibody* to HIV-1." (Epitope, Inc. U.S. License #1133.)

So what you do here is first *presume* that samples reactive on ELISA and WB are positive for *antibodies*, and since the CDC says so (well, they are going to say so on August 14, 1987; see below), you get to further *presume* that persons with antibodies are infected. Logically, then, all persons reactive on ELISA and WB should likewise be *presumed* to be infected (i.e., If A = B, and B = C, then A = C; with the exception that in the above equation, there are NO equal signs).

JULY 23, 1987: Researchers/Burroughs Welcome Corporation publish the results of their clinical trial demonstrating "AZT administration can decrease mortality and the frequency of opportunistic infections in a selected group of subjects with AIDS or AIDS-related complex, at least over the 8 to 24 weeks of observation in this study." (*N Engl J Med* July 23, 1987; 317: 185-91).

AUGUST 14, 1987: Without reference to any scientific study, or any previous report from the CDC, the CDC announces: "*The presence of antibody indicates current infection*, though many infected persons may have minimal or no clinical evidence of disease for years." (CDC. "Perspectives in disease prevention and health promotion public health service guidelines for counseling and antibody testing to prevent HIV infection and AIDS." *MMWR* August 14, 1987; 36(31): 509-15.) Gone is "presumed," "considered," "for public health purposes," etc. Gone is any distinction between "blood donors" and "high risk;" between "asymptomatic" and "symptomatic."

It is important to note that the designated mission of the CDC is public disease surveillance, education, and prevention. Here they are implicitly setting standards for medical practice. More precisely, they are establishing standards for medical practice without any scientific justification. Why the FDA (our consumer protection agency) choose to completely ignore this blatant violation of medical ethics remains an enigma. This is particularly the case when only four months earlier, the FDA warned, "*The significance of antibodies in an asymptomatic individual is not known*" (Susan Cruzan. *FDA News* 4/30/1987; P87-11). Without doubt, August 14, 1987 will ultimately come to be known as the day modern science came to an end.

The debt of gratitude toward the many people who made it possible for this material to see the light of day—starting in 1987 and culminating with this book—is deeper than I am able to express. The personal cost to each person—scientist and civilian alike—who became part of the vast human chain of this (to say the least) unpopular story, was immeasurable. We see only shards of it in this text, but the reality is that this "uncensored history" was kept alive by people who in most cases took very serious blows to their careers and lives. The generosity and courage they showed me over the years—the time they took to explain, document, and explain again the various things I was perpetually asking them·about— was limitless. They always helped me convert my "question marks into exclamation marks," as my friend Peter Olsen so beautifully puts it.

I hope you trust that the metaphor of the ants is incidental, in this passage of Tomas Transtromer:

"And each man-ant brought his own little stroke to add to the big engraving, there was no proper center, but everything was alive."

Celia Farber
New York City
2006

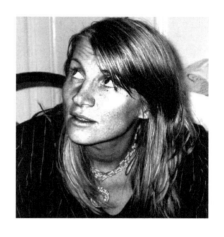

From 1987 to 1997, CELIA FARBER wrote and edited *SPIN* magazine's AIDS column, "Words From The Front." She has also written for many magazines and newspapers, including *Esquire, Rolling Stone, Gear, Salon*, and *Harper's*. She lives in New York City.